KABOOMER

THRIVING *and* STRIVING
INTO YOUR NINETIES

DAVID EMERSON FROST

Disclaimer

All material in this book and/or on associated sites (wellpastforty.com, babykaboomers.com, stamininety.com) is provided for your information and potential use only, and may not be considered as medical advice, nutritional advice, or nutritional instruction. No personal action or inaction should be taken solely due to the contents of this book and/or associated information. Readers are advised to consult health professionals on any matter relating to their health or wellbeing.

Well Past Forty
——— PUBLISHING ———

Well Past Forty LLC
17164 Libertad Drive
San Diego, CA. 92127
USA
wellpastforty.com
info@wellpastforty.com
ISBN: 978-0578-628547 (print)
ISBN: 978-0578-628554(ebook)
Ordering Information:
Special discounts are available on quantity purchases by corporations, associations, and others. For details, contact: info@wellpastforty.com or +18589253895

TABLE OF CONTENTS

What's a KABOOMER, Anyway?

A KABOOMER is an ageless "never quit tryin'" Dolly Parton. A KABOOMER is a "boss" Bruce Springsteen. Most importantly, a KABOOMER could be **you**.

- Do you ask, "Why not?" rather than question "Why?" when opportunity arises?

- Do you stretch for golden rings as "little extras" in your circle of life?

- Do you tell friends and strangers that "I may get older, but I do not get old!"?

- Do you wither not, eat clean, move, stretch, and get your earned Z's?

- Do you build your physical 401(k) account to live better as you live longer?

If not you, who? If not soon, when will you start to KA-BOOM?

Like a Phoenix

All baby boomers remember that fateful Tuesday morning, September 11, 2001. I was in London for business, wincing from my recent herniated disk and sciatica. There I heard a BBC announcer state, "The skyline of New York City has changed forever." To paraphrase Kris Kristofferson's 1970s anthem: "Why us and why me, Lord?"

When world-changing events happen, we ask ourselves: Can our nation rise again like a phoenix? Now we know that answer is YES.

Personal setbacks happen as well. Could I be a phoenix; rising and healing after my own injury and spinal fusion? Now I know that this answer is also YES.

By 2002, I had established new fitness habits to deal with my physical challenges. When medically cleared after spinal fusion surgery, I found my mid-life substitute for distance running. Sure, even now, I miss my runner's highs, my "sub-6" mile runs, and 2:56 marathon finishes. (And I would like to miss the frisks of my metallic back by TSA airport screeners.)

Then I found my purpose and became a Master Fitness Trainer, an elite master's rower and crew mentor, and a "KA-BOOMER Koach" who can now share actionable lessons learned with you.

You may have chosen (or been given) this book because you face your own life challenges, setbacks, or obstacles—if so, read on! If not, also read on to help you avoid those issues when they arise as speed bumps on your fitness and wellness travels. Physical challenge(s)? Let's also acknowledge diabetes, MS, sleep disorders, asthma, cancer, and many other speed bumps that can impede our journeys if we let them. I am a cancer survivor, and you may be a blessed survivor as well. Do you have unhealthy body mass issues or metabolic syndrome abnormalities?

Carpe Diem. Form your health habits to shake those life-sapping, deadly conditions as best you can.

KABOOMER: *Thriving and Striving into your 90s* asserts that age 70 can be your new 40. And that 90 years young is a perfect partying age. Yes, I offer solid evidence that you can face aging effects head-on and **slow** aging processes for both your body and your mind. Yes, you can maintain lean skeletal muscle and party past 90. You can stay flexible and balanced to avert deadly falls. You can eat clean and construct your very own "geroprotection"[1] anti-aging policy. You can deal better with the little and not-so-little stresses of life. And you can enjoy your rightful restorative and restful sleep.[2] Yes, you can!

Have a look at titular themes for determined folks who intend to KABOOM:

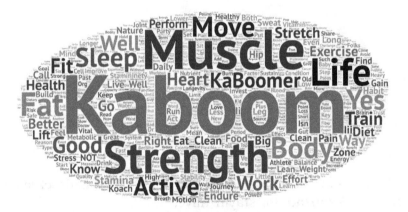

Details behind our word-cloud themes and I (as your KABOOMER Koach) will *habitually* help you add years to your life *and* quality life to your years. With my decades of experience and expertise, I can show you seven ways to party past 90 in protracted and productive KABOOMER ways. This tailored wellness project is for those of us born between 1946 and 1964—like Dolly Parton, Bruce Springsteen, former Governor Arnold Schwarzenegger—and most importantly, like **you**.

Trust me. Rise up, party on like these two of our partying peers.

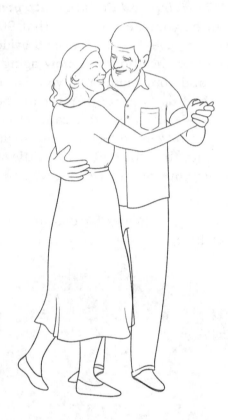

Let's begin our KABOOMER journey with its bedrock component, **Stamina,** for stayin' alive.

CHAPTER 1

Stamina —Your Key to Stayin' Alive

Now you are ready to shift gears to become a bona fide KA-BOOMER. As you shift 'em, your journey is predicated on a strong foundation of exercise and stamina. Exercise **can be as effective as drugs**. Does that resonate with you as it does with me?

> "Our results show that...exercise can be as effective as what is accomplished today with drugs."—Kerry Stewart, Ed.D., professor of medicine at The Johns Hopkins University School of Medicine

Dwell on this JHU professor's assertion, please. An effective alternative to "polypharmacy" (multiple drug prescriptions) is exercise. This assumes that you are averse to becoming a older polydrug user—like ten million boomer peers. Don't look for any workout tips just yet. *KABOOMER: Thriving and Striving into your 90s* is topped with trusted tips to improve your health and longevity. First, let us examine Why.

Why? For improved stamina, naturally. Build up your stamina, then prepare to dance and live large, with fewer pharmaceuticals in your system.

"Regular exercise extended the lives in every group that we examined in our study—normal weight, overweight, or obese."—Steven Moore, Ph.D., National Cancer Institute

Life Extension! Sure, being of normal weight and lean body composition is healthier than being overweight or obese. However, it is more critical that readers are *stayin' alive (longer) by building their health and endurance.* Do **not** stress over the man or woman you see in the mirror today. Positive changes to your body fat and body silhouette and to your vital physical accounts will follow with endured exercise (and diet, and sleep, and...).

Stamina Is Currency in Your Physical Bank Account

"Pay yourself first."—John Paul DeJoria, founder of Patròn and Paul Mitchell

Let's equate your *fiscal* retirement model for your golden years with your new *physical* banking model for stamina and KABOOMER vitality.

Retirement: You paid yourself first in your professional life with pre-tax or IRA investments that you confidently tucked away for your golden years. Some of you, like me, are there now. These fiscal resources are tangible stashes in secure bank accounts that you can tap for future wants and needs in life. These time-valued monies can be a principal factor in your livelihood and quality of life, yes?

Reserves: Now, shift your sight to your *physical* bank vaults. You can and should build up, over time, reserves of capacity that give you the *stamina* to survive and *subvert senescence.* With these 401(k) reserves – you will KABOOM. *Senescence* is a romantic language expression for **bodily deterioration,** which is *not* romantic.

To KABOOM is to **offset** and **oppose** senescence with sustained motion and a bit of sweat.

Stamina is a person's innate and/or acquired ability to sustain effort, as measured by time or distance. So...a KABOOM-ER *sustains* effort by breathing and moving at a quick pace for a half-hour or longer almost every day of every week. He or she thereby *slow burns* stored energy (glycogen or fat) via the body's amazing aerobic systems. He or she thereby gains *stamina* for *stayin' alive.*

The Fountain of Youth?! I do not know of any fast fix, miracle method, or mysterious element to build your bedrock stamina for longevity. If there ever was such a thing, it probably drowned in the mythical Fountain of Youth, which Ponce de León never found. Jesting aside, there is, *without* a doubt, a Fountain of Youth in your body. It just needs *your low intensity effort for at least 30 minutes on most days* so you can generate sweat to trigger those amazing anti-aging processes in your KABOOMER body. Try it, you'll like it. And then try it longer and better. Make it a habit and you'll love livin' large and partying on – just like those two KABOOMERs cutting a rug on our book cover!

As you'll read in other segments, it is your very own "quick" pace at effort that matters; **not** the quick pace of anyone else. You are a unique physical specimen with your very own **athlete** within.

Are you an athlete?

You bet you are. There is no doubt. None other than Bill Bowerman, the inventor of the original Nike waffle trainer shoe, advised: "If you have a body, you *are* an athlete."

I share again: your body, on its enduring and vital journey of stayin' alive, is unique. So is your unique "slow burning" of stored energy. Your bespoke physical bank vault can and should gain value over time to arrest, or to subvert, cellular aging. When you build your physical bank account as an athlete, you will gain **stamininety.**

While each KABOOMER's physical bank is different, his/her journey signposts are the same. Here they are:

Build physical *stamina* with these healthy habits:

- Sweat for three *or more* hours each week.
- Sustain effort in your best heart rate zone to load up your physical bank vault.
- Know the answer to "*Why* should I move?" and "What's in it for *me*?"
- Challenge your left ventricle and amazing lungs to pump you up.
- Listen to your marvelous body; it will tell you when to sustain effort and when to rest. With practice, you will recognize the signs when it is talking to you.
- Be safe.

How?

Ascribe to this investment metaphor as your physical principle to build KABOOMER **stamina**. *You only draw working capital from what you have deposited in your physical bank account.*

Or, as Muddy Waters sang, "You can't spend what you ain't got; you can't lose what you ain't never had." You can only tap the endurance capability that you have earned and deposited.

Hold this thought: Please invest *at least two-thirds* of your endurance or stamina workouts every week, every year, at your own *low intensity zone* of effort! (You'll shortly learn what your appropriate heart rate is.) Those nominal weekly investments of about three hours a week may well add years to your life. Should you not trust me (yet), do trust what the National Cancer Institute has to say.[3]

I'm not a gambler. Yet if I was, I'd like those anti-aging odds, whatever my current body composition was. *Yes— even if we carry extra fat—we extend our lives when we regularly move to sweat.* KABOOM! I move a lot to improve my odds. I want you to move as well.

Your Favorite Radio Station—WIFM—and a Fave DJ

> "We are put on this earth to have a good time. This makes other people feel good. And the cycle continues." —Legendary American radio DJ Wolfman Jack

What's in it for me (WIFM)? Your "what" is having more good times and lasting *longer* in your cycle!

Regardless of your current body profile, take note and then act because *motion is medicine.* Your cyclical motion, at the right intensity and over time, slows down the aging processes that sedentary boomers, like Joe and Sally Six Pack, experience in their Act III's. The "what" is that you can add quality years to your life, and you can put quality life into your years. **Move to Sweat** on most days and enjoy more parties—longer! Move even if your "guy" profile resembles Joe's six pack (below) with his evident and unhealthy "apple" shape (more about apples and pears later). Yes, ladies, a similar challenge is on Jill Six Pack's table too.

Joe Six Pack

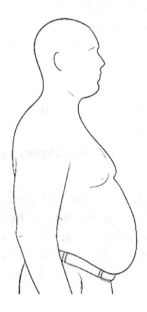

Wolfman Jack's Station Break: *"When blood and O_2 don't flow, you don't go!"*

Now back to your WIFM broadcast. Note: We'll delve into why you need to generate sweat. When sweating, you trigger cellular repair and growth. No Sweat, no Growth. Read on to learn more.

Feel the Beat for Stamininety

Your Koach asserts this: your knowledge of your resting heart rate, maximum heart rate, and recovery rate after exercise is ***imperative*** to proper physical banking.

Cookie-cutter heart rate models may fit the general boomer populace, but they may not fit you. They assuredly do not fit me! Feel *your* beat!

Feeling your beat(s) is *not* a trivial pursuit. If you exercise in a heart-rate zone that's too high, you'll be exhausted and potentially in physical danger. But if your zone is too low, you won't develop the base fitness and stamina for stayin' alive longer.

Get *into your zone* at the right heart rate and perceived exertion level as you move to sweat and then recover. Whether you establish your own "cardio" zones or seek assistance from a peer or pro, you need to train *in your zone* for reasons you will soon learn.

As a starter, you can estimate maximum heart rate with this cookie cutter guesstimate:

220 heart beats per minute (bpm) minus your age in calendar years

Example: A reasonably healthy 65-year-old female could use this basic formula to guesstimate her maximum training heart rate of 220 minus 65, or 155 beats per minute. Of course, she should get her MD's permission to safely elevate her heart rate, to gain stamina and to glisten. This starting number is a pretty good estimate for most baby boomers to use.

A "nominal" heart rate (HR) zone for this female is about 110 beats per minute to build stamina over time. She can move a bit slower if her heart rate *still* exceeds 50 percent of that 155-bpm estimate—or 78 beats per minute (BPM)—for about thirty minutes. I leave a marker for moving faster over time, as walking speed *is* a valid estimator of your longevity.

Perceived exertion? If she can speak short sentences without breathing heavily as she moves, her exertion levels are at a "best heart rate zone" to gain stamina. She might ask, "How 'bout those damn Yankees?" as she walks briskly, or bikes, or pauses at the lap pool wall. If she *can't* comfortably share sentence fragments during her activity, her exertions are *above* the capacity-building zone for her ticker. I kid you not!

Invest time in low intensity, chatting activities to build **your** *physical bank account.*

This training zone of *50 to 66 percent* of your estimated maximum heart rate to build stamina is vitally important if you intend to live long and well. By the way, *the conversational zone for exertion and HR* (50 to 66 percent of max heart rate) works well for folks of all ages.

KABOOMERs may well have, or may well develop, cardiovascular and respiratory systems that are better fitted to another estimator to move at the "right" exertion levels to build their physical bank account. I just shared that a "vanilla" 220 age estimation method above doesn't fit my activity. If it did, my maximum estimated heart rate would be 220 bpm at 67 years of age, or a maximal rate of 163 beats per minute (in 2020). My *measured* maximum heart rate is 180 bpm. My outlier beats are an illustration for using the "tool that fits you" to move and sweat in the most beneficial way. So, an initial estimate of 82-110 bpm that fits many folks is a tad low for my own stamininety efforts. Remember: you <u>are unique!</u>

Or Try This

I use an alternate "Karvonen" heart rate estimating formula (208 beats per minute minus 0.7 times my current resting heart rate) as a maximal training rate estimate.[5] Then I plan my stayin' alive (stamina) workouts based on that maximum heart rate estimate.

Note: Most of us *don't* need a formal stress test to peg our maximum heart rate. Finders, keepers.

Find Your Personal Stamina Zone

Here is *your 1-2-3* approach to move at the *right* intensity to build physical 401(k) reserves.

Have Fun at Number One

Call **Zone 1** your (current) training heart rate zone in which you can converse comfortably without heavy breathing as you move. Note: I say "current" as your zones should favorably change as you progress on your stamina journey.

This Zone marks your approximate activity or training to maintain a rate of 50 to 66 percent of your current maximum estimated heart rate. Think of it as your cruise control—at *half power* exertion to tour cross-country and enjoy your scenic journey.

A quick example: A KABOOMER's maximum estimated heart rate, at present, (as it should favorably change) is 165 beats per minute.

Sustained walking, jogging, or other activities that "burn fat" build your aerobic capacity and let you converse at "low" intensity. Yet still *sweat* with your heart pulsing between 82 and 110 beats per minute.

Yes, there are many web or smart phone applications to help you with your own heart rate (HR) monitoring effort. Yet your luddite scribe encourages you to learn how to get "in the zone" in an ol' fashioned way.

Listen to your body and count your arterial thumps for ten seconds, then multiply by 6 to acquire your "real time" heart rate. You can feel your pulse at your carotid (neck), brachial (wrist), or femoral (groin) arterial spots. *I personally skip femoral (groin) artery checks for HR when I am in public settings.* But you count your ticks where you wanna count them. Know your body! Example: If you count 19 beats in a ten-second timed window, your real-time heart rate is 114 bpm.

Here is what Koach Dave calls your **80/20 Stamina Rule:**

Invest up to **80 percent** of your stamina efforts in your training Zone 1. As you are ready and cleared, you can and should invest up to **20 percent** of your stamina time in higher HR Zones 2 and 3. Only then... and with these notations...

1. As you get fitter on your stamina journey, your stronger left ventricle muscle can pump more blood with stayin' alive nutrients per each beat.

2. Your maximum heart rate is a function of genetics, general health, and age. Our maximum heart rate usually drops for most of our adult lives. This is one reason why younger athletes may outperform us. Yet KABOOMERs do their best with inherited "cardio" system and physical 401(k) capacity, yes?

3. As you get fitter on your stamina journey, your recovery time after bumping up your heart rate drops too! This is one mark of stamininety—*heart rate recovery*. Stayin' Alive.

Zone 2 Beats

Let us examine a **Zone 2** for your stamina/endurance efforts to subvert cellular aging. This middle beat zone is gauged when you're breathing heavily, and you *cannot* sustain normal conversation while moving or exerting in some way. (Yes, moving and heavy breathing between your bed sheets counts.) You *cannot* sustain activity in this heart rate zone as you can for lower intensity Zone 1 endurance efforts. We just aren't built for that. Zone 2 is a *higher* aerobic zone for a nominal 20 minutes of exertion. *If* you surpass your aerobic threshold, *then* your amazing body can shift to its primordial anaerobic energy system for short periods. Stay tuned for more about anaerobic efforts. For now, just know that if you're panting and breathing heavily, you're likely at, or exceeding, your capacity to sustain your aerobic performance in that lower Zone 1. This Zone 2 effort is fine for short exertion spells of up to ~ 20 minutes, once or twice a week.

Zone 2 exertion **can** be sustained for "mid running distances" of 5 to 10 kilometers when you become an elite, superbly conditioned endurance athlete. That time, speed, distance rule of thumb works for *other* sports or activities too. **Think of high aerobic performance for shorter periods** than you would likely exert for longer periods of time in Zone 1. Most baby boomers are not ready for high aerobic performance like this. KABOOMERs are ready! Getting in this second stamina Zone be a climactic heart-thumpin', heavy breathin' run, or bike, or row, or swim. Or a get-lucky, go all the way home run.

- Approximate Zone 2 heart rates are from **67 to 80 percent** of your current maximum heart rate for exertions.

For our same example 65-year-old (with an estimated maximum training heart rate of 165 bpm), her Zone 2 performance for heart rate *ranges* from 110 bpm to 132 bpm. Sure, it is very good for her, and for us, to invest stamina efforts in Zone 2, up to *20 percent* of one's total cardio time. My abacus shows that if you invest 180 minutes per week in stamina efforts; you can invest about *36 minutes* of Zone 2 effort in your HR baseline. If you endure *more* minutes per week, your invested Zone 2 times increase too. I am blessed to invest at least five hours (300 minutes) on my weekly stamina journey, so I get into my Zone 2 for one hour (60 minutes) each training week. That's my 80/20 KABOOMER rule for Stayin' Alive. That is *your* rule too.

Important point: You should *not* invest too much time here in Zone 2. Honest. You don't build up that physical 401(k) principal with extra time or effort in higher intensity Zones 2 (or 3). Plus, you need time for your body to refresh and restore. *Don't* skip your R&R! *Don't* go too hard, too often. Repeat, repeat; **do** invest lotsa time in your Zone 1 HR efforts. Add a little quality time in Zone 2 and wait, wait Zone 3 for stayin' alive heart rates. Trust the experts like your Koach. KABOOM.

KABOOM in Zone 3, briefly

Zone 3 is our *short-term* elevated heart rate (HR) zone. A top zone in which you're breathing intensely and have *no* desire to converse while rapidly moving and/or working darned hard. This "high" intensity zone can be thought of as your *sprint* zone. Yes, your body's high aerobic efforts may hand off to your *anaerobic* energy system at some point in such intense Zone 3 activity.

Our anaerobic system provides uber-power, but only for short periods before we need to replenish and recover. Think of the world's fastest man, Usain Bolt. His eponymous sprint velocity *six seconds* from his starting blocks was 27+ miles per hour. That bolt velocity is greased millennial lightning. Yet it is also the point at which he slowed down because his system (or ours) *can't* sustain a high anaerobic level of effort for longer. I'll bet a nickel that I might sustain effort and compete credibly with the world's fastest man, **if** an event distance of my choosing was long enough. I'm a long-haul KABOOMER. You should build your long-haul capacity too!

Our high intensity, aerobic red zone for heart rate rises to 90 percent or more of your current "max" cardiovascular capacity. *Rojo!* Our exemplar lady with her current training heart rate maximum of 165 beats per minute, pegs her Zone 3 rating at about 148 bpm. THUMP, rapidly THUMP. Thumpin' and breathin' heavily with a short burst of power, *when you are ready* for these all-out intervals. (Remember to check with your health professional before you hit your top end or "red zone.")

Swedes have a name for steady endurance periods interspersed with intense red zones or "speed plays." "Fartleks" are what they call these interspersed Zone 1 or 2 aerobics and high intensity Zone 3 periods. I've been known to call my intense red-zone experiences something else of the four-letter variety.

- Even supremely fit KABOOMERs work "only" about 20 percent or at most 30 % of their total stamina time in Zones 2 and 3. This is **exercise science**. Remember, sprinter Bolt *only* bolts for ~ 6 seconds at his unworldly top end before slowing! Remember your long-haul, prosperous 80/20 party rule!

Live Well and Prosper

As a KABOOMER, you have, or will have a "real" wellness age or a "gym age" that is lower than your chronological age. This lower "gym" age is truly one that you can celebrate. Post a note:

KABOOMERs have measured "gym ages" aka "fitness ages"[7] that are *lower* than their chronological years.

You can and should be proud of your notably *low* gym age. I am! Stamina in my physical accounts is helping me live better and prosper longer. How about you?

Stamina does have a positive impact on longevity and wellness. I promise!

Sure, we acknowledge nasty flip sides of life that can prematurely close our physical 401(k)s. Hereditary heart disease, smoking, and heavy drinking can subvert boomer or KABOOMER intentions and physical actions. You can also avoid using seat belts and you can live in solitude (lacking social connections) if you choose to accelerate your Grim

Reaper's visit. Sure, you could have an untimely accident or fall a victim to cancer as a hard punch to your gut.

Here's your upbeat KABOOMER counterpunch:

Your stamina and endurance mitigate or remediate diabetes, heart, and lung conditions.

A stamina counterpunch equates to your *extended* life and your *quality* of life, for work and play. Stamina soundly means that you move and sweat often. Paint a personal portrait of *life and breath and sweat!* Motion **is** medicine. Motion is a precursor to partying past 90. No, I'm *not* senile as I offer this!

A Smidgen of Science

A couch potato or a dormant desk jockey suffers a daily *decay* of cellular vitality without bodily repair, recovery, and growth. Regular endurance (and strength) activities **can** slow biological aging or "senescence", period. Experts, like those at the National Institutes of Health[6] , state, "... intermittent fasting, physical exercise, intake of antioxidants such as resveratrol and curcumin have shown **considerable** promise for improving function in aging."

Please note related promises of diet, lifestyle, and exercise.

The more scientists research and analyze *performance versus age*, the more positive findings they document for stamina efforts that **subvert senescence.** (This big word—**senescence**—is related to both *senile* and *senate*.) By moving often and vigorously enough to sweat, we stimulate our cardio-respiratory pipes and energy pathway systems. Did I mention stamininety? Remember Forrest Gump, who ran and ran? He had it. Or remember our generational balladeer, Bruce Springsteen, who has it. The Boss' "Born to Run" anthem resonates with me. Resonant, though I'd modify his words a smidgen: "Baby, we were born to **move and sweat.**"

Name your motion. Just make those motions long enough to sweat, whether it's yard work, cycling, swimming, striding, or taking turns in Cupid's court.

Let's get it on. Change things up. Be different on your journey, as my shirtsleeve relative wrote.

"I took the one less traveled by,

And that has made all the difference."
—Robert Frost

Are you locked and loaded to improve chances for a longer, quality-filled life? If so, take the road *not* traveled by *most* boomers. Make a difference for your family members, friends, and yourself by living longer and living better. Not the poetic type? Then ponder and act on lifting lyrics by Led Zeppelin ("Stairway to Heaven"). Let me be your piper.

Do you strive to invest that *little bit extra to be extraordinary?* If so, this book provides your toolkit to gain that 'lil bit extra. However, if you are content to live your days as an average "Jack or Jill," please pass this guidebook to a friend or loved one. Let me be clear: KABOOMERs are different from baby boomers. Many of those living and dying differences stem from our individual plans and successful habits and actions. So, let's codify differences between ordinary "them" and 'lil bit extra "**us**."

Let's start our comparison with a Knock-Knock.

Knock-Knock.
Who's There?
A baby boomer and a KABOOMER.
A baby boomer and KABOOMER Who?
A boomer who may take two pills at a time and a KABOOMER who takes steps two at a time!

Twenty boomer and **KABOOMER** comparisons should stimulate your extraordinary thoughts and actions to live longer and better.

Your Koach picks just one from our summary lists to emphasize that 'lil bit extra: Body Profile, which is germane to that Knock-knock.

An ordinary boomer likely has a HIGHER, unhealthy waist-to-hip ratio than an extraordinary KABOOMER. With that bigger boomer waist may come a cluster of unhealthy conditions called **metabolic syndrome**, and quite possibly **non-alcoholic fatty liver disease** (NAFLD). Oy!

Traits of Ordinary Baby Boomers vs. Extraordinary KABOOMERs

Ordinary Traits of Baby Boomers
1. Resides in the lower half of our boomer demographic for wellness and fitness.
2. Likely to die before, or just reach, the Social Security Administration's actuarial life expectancy.
www.ssa.gov/oact/STATS/table4c6.html
3. Unhealthy apple-shaped body profile (higher waist-to-hip ratio).
4. Sub-normal or normal gym age, meaning that physical performance matches chronological age.
5. Nominal sentiments for seven elements (7S) of long and healthy lives:
Strength *"Please help me, I can't lift this carry-on case."*
Stability *"I trip and fall more than I should."*
Stamina *"I'm often too tired to enjoy activities with family and friends."*
Stretching *"I can't seem to reach for things like I used to."*
Stressing *"Life just gets me down."*
Sleep *"No matter what I try, I don't get restful sleep."*

Sustenance *"I just eat what I like, and fast casual dining is okay."*	
6. "Faster than normal" or "normal" aging equals early senescence of bodily cells.	
7. Likely to suffer early loss of skeletal muscles (known as sarcopenia).	
8. Chronic internal inflammation/oxidative damages from life stressors.	
9. Suffers from unhealthy metabolic syndrome.	
10. Below average testosterone levels "T" (without supplementation).	
11. Marks time, content with status quo of generational peers.	
12. Accepts life's circumstances.	
13. Slips off the wellness wagon of good habits "too often."	
14. Content to be in the "norm."	
15. Lives to eat.	
16. Asks what happened? Or watches what happens.	
17. Has nil or low motivation to become a KABOOMER with a 'lil bit extra.	
18. Yes, but I don't have time.	
19. Yearns for the happy or happier days of the past.	
20. Leaves the best that life offers for others and becomes a burden to the next generation.	

Extraordinary Traits of KABOOMERs

1. Reside in the upper half of our boomer demographic for wellness and fitness performances.	
2. Likely to live beyond the Social Security Administration's actuarial life expectancy.	
www.ssa.gov/oact/STATS/table4c6.html	

3.	Healthier pear-shaped body profile (lower waist-to-hip ratio).
4.	Superior gym age, meaning that physical performance matches a younger chronological age.
5.	Nominal sayings and sentiments for seven elements (7S) of long and healthy lives are:

Strength *"I can lift this carry-on case for you."*

Stability *"I rarely trip or fall. I know that sitting is the new smoking."*

Stamina *"I'm ever ready to enjoy activities with my family and friends."*

Stretching *"I can reach that brass ring just like in my younger days."*

Stressing *"Neither little nor big things in life get me down."*

Sleep *"I regularly get my restorative sleep."*

Sustenance *"I eat cleanly out of habit about 80 percent of the time."*

6.	"Slower than normal" aging, without tendency for early senescence of bodily cells.
7.	Far less likely to suffer early loss of skeletal muscles (sarcopenia)
8.	Mitigates internal inflammation/oxidative damages from life stressors.
9.	Avoids or markedly reduces effects of unhealthy metabolic syndrome.
10.	Above average testosterone levels "T" (without supplementation).
11.	Makes time; rarely content with status quo of generational peers.
12.	Makes the best of life, each, and every day.

13. Stays on the wellness wagon of good habits "80 percent of the time."
14. Discontent with "normalcy."
15. Eats to live longer and better.
16. Makes things happen!
17. Sustains motivation to party past 90 as a KABOOMER!
18. Yes, AND I make time to leverage life's opportunities.
19. Earns many more happy days ahead.
20. Enjoys the best that life offers and stays independent past 90.

Notes:

1. This table provides subjective limits rather than objective performance and behavior metrics in our Medicare days.

2. Hold the thought that *motion is medicine,* no matter how modified that motion is.

Let's acknowledge and address special sub-populations which may need modified motion. Diabetics, folks with skeletal issues, those with nature-provided or mishap-driven limitations, and those living with asthma, multiple sclerosis (MS), or cerebral palsy (CP), or Parkinson's disease are all included in our boomer demographic.

I have *not* seen a valid study result or document that advises these sub-populations to live as couch potatoes. To limit their motion, and/or throw in the towel and deny living their dolce vita as best they can. Play the hand that you were dealt. MOVING (per approval of your medical and health professionals) until you sweat is *rarely* contraindicated.

3. What is that 'lil bit extra in an aggregate sense?

Eat well and clean. Laugh often. Chill. Figure out how to get those credibly recommended 420 minutes or more of restful and restorative sleep[8] on most nights. Each KABOOMER builds a physical 401(k) from which to tap resources to "party past 90 and to love the one you're with" (thank you, Stephen Stills).

In ensuing pages, I offer my experiential journey and lessons to help you with your own journey to thrive and strive. I add valid recommendations for your better and longer lives. Steps which are both possible and plausible. Worthy habits which are within your grasp, which build on your stamina bedrock, and which make you a rock star for living long and well. It can be done. It should be done. And I hope that you are one bad a@# KABOOMER that will do it!

If you have *already* earned your chops as a card-carrying KABOOMER, listen to my virtual applause for your low "gym age" and prospects for stamininety. Please read on still ...you will still benefit from useful hints and hacks for your journey. And you'll likely share with others, as TED talks do, that these KABOOMER ideas *are* worth sharing.

Unless you can walk on water, you are probably a bit short of perfection. As for me, I fall well short of perfection, as my sainted bride of 44 years (in 2020) may mention.

Here is the big idea, and what follows is your interrelated action plan to build your physical 401(k) account. Your account for stayin' alive. Your physical portfolio for thriving and striving into your 90s.

Your KABOOMER's Big Idea and Action Plan with Seven Elements

Note: These six ringed elements for KABOOMER health intersect at our "don't worry", STRESS *NOT* center of successful "7S" journeys.

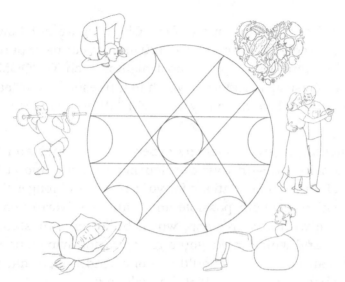

Start at any clock position, and then repeat after your KA-BOOMER Koach:

Strength, Stability, Stamina, Stretching, Sustenance, Sleep, and Stress (Not).

Let's use these seven embracing elements as your healthy habit-formers to party past 90!

Folks, I haven't found proof of a magical elixir from the Fountain of Youth or Madison Avenue. I haven't found a "pixie dust" pill, elixir or potion to mystically eliminate belly fat (aka muffin top) over which some boomers obsess. If anyone knows of a cure-all detoxification smoothie to help you drop 30 years from your gym age—*please* get on a TED talk to spread that great idea. Till then, take small, positive steps. Till then, *form lasting habits* for motion as medicine, with sweat, sleep, and stability (to avoid falls). Chill, socialize, and don't sweat the small hassles of life. And eat as if your long life depended on it...

Ready? Set? Go and KABOOM as the last guy or gal dancin'. Build your physical 401(k) account reserves now. Start with habitual small steps and your journey will be longer and more enjoyable.

CHAPTER 2

Motion is Medicine

Congratulations for passing "Go" in our key **Stamina for Stayin' Alive** introduction. You will now learn that *little bit extra* for your bedrock of longevity and enhanced quality of life. A literal difference between ordinary and extraordinary is that *'lil bit extra*. All that's left to do is your 'lil bit extra to sustain your habit-forming movement to sweat at least 30 minutes on most days.

On your mark...your innate or acquired ability to sustain effort, as measured by time or distance is **stamininety**.

Get set...with motioned KABOOMER checkmarks:

Move to sweat for three or more hours each week.

Determine your bespoke heart rate (HR) training zones.

Answer your own "Why should I move?" and "What's in this for me?" queries.

Challenge your left ventricle and amazing lungs.

Listen to your marvelous body and its feedback signs.

Be safe on your sustained successful journey.

Go! You are that special person with *upgraded* stamina. Your return on investment (ROI) for sweat and heart rate *is* a prolific physical 401(k), and you can have a blast while earning it. I don't claim that adding years to your boomer life and ensuring quality years in your boomer life is an easy venture. I don't offer miracle cures or expedient solutions. Nor do I suggest that we can completely suppress family and personal histories of illness or lack of fitness. Life does happen; KABOOMER stamina is not an ironclad guarantee for longevity or quality of life. One may recall that the gent who chronicled his joy of running, James Fixx, succumbed to heart problems which "ran in his family." Yet, his quality of life lived was joyful. Your author certainly sports more warts than beauty marks. So, I joyfully move to sweat to subvert senescence.

Agreed! Most of "us" 75 million American boomers have slight or not-so-slight imperfections. Supreme Court Justice Antonin Scalia admonished us to "play the hand we were dealt." Yes, he played his card hand with smoking as a personal choice. Perhaps his demise was related to that "Marlboro Man" habit. Surely, both nature and nurture affect medical condition or strength, profile look, longevity, or stamina. Studies suggest that 5-10% of one's risk for developing diseases like diabetes comes from your genes (DNA). If you were dealt that diabolic hand, do your best to fit into your jeans...

Example: You have type 1 or type 2 diabetes. Most *diabetic* adults **can** benefit from prudent moving and sweating (carefully, under advisement of medical professionals) and clean eating to keep their waist to hip ratios as healthy as possible.

You just acquired a working knowledge of **"1–2–3"** training zones for your monitored heart rate and sweat to build stamina. You appreciated, though it seems counterintuitive, that most of your stamina efforts should be at "low" intensity heart rates. **Keeping your heart rate at two-thirds or less of your calculated maximum heart rate** for most workouts is a **key** to building capacity. Keep that **80/20 rule** for stamina efforts alive. Trust your Koach that this is true. Your endured efforts in this "low" heart rate (HR) zone builds capacity to sustain "cardio" effort.

Cardio 101

It's time to entertain you with factoids about your cardio-vascular and cardio-pulmonary systems. Both are vital systems that allow us to extend our super-charged KABOOMER capacity.

- Each of us has about 60,000 miles of pipes to transport oxygen and nutrients to our many billions of cells.

- A single red blood cell takes *about a minute* for a complete "lap" while we are at rest.

- Endured sweaty efforts truly stimulate: 1. the expansion of your circulatory mileage; 2. the number of mitochondria (those micro-power generators in all our cells); and 3. your lungs' exchange capacity.

- Complementing these vital circulation highways are your lesser known and studied lymphatic waste collection and disposal highways. These disposal systems are not glamorous, yet they are also vital[9]!

- Any 90-year-old with a resting heart rate of 70 beats per minute has had more than 3 billion heart beats. A KABOOMER should have many *more* beats left at that point. Thump, KABOOM.

  - *How important is your monitored heart rate?* Uber-important. Feel your Beat! *Count your ticks often, starting when your feet hit the deck after a nightly restful sleep.*

- Favorable brain-changing[10] effects of your stamina efforts are well-documented and validated for KABOOMER protection, function, and feeling good! A single workout increases your level of "happy" neurotransmitters, like dopamine, serotonin, and noradrenaline. Boosted mood. A single workout can improve your ability to focus attention. A single workout will improve your reaction times. You are going to be faster at catching that cup of Starbucks that falls off the counter."

"Movement to sweat is your super-charged physical 401(k)." – Dr. Wendy Suzuki

More superchargers:

- Telo-whats? Unless you are an astronaut on extended space travel, the best way to lengthen your DNA caps called *telomeres*[11] is to exercise. You'll read more about the importance of telomeres as lengthened end caps on your DNA strands.

- Lungs have the approximate surface area of a tennis court in which to exchange inbound oxygen (O_2) and outbound carbon dioxide (CO_2). A tennis court is **2,800** square feet.

- A biochemical bottom line of stamina effort is this: "Just keep breathing."[12]

- Your combined exhalations of water vapor and skin-cooling sweat loss can exhaust 2-3 liters of water daily (not counting exercise). Be safe and drink water before you get thirsty

  - Each of us was born with 2–4 billion sweat cells near the surface of our skin (except in our ears and on our lips, though I think my lips sweat if I have excess wasabi on my sashimi).

  - The principal byproduct of your fat-burning is water vapor. Yup!

  - Sweating too little can be dangerous and even life-threatening!

- "Sweat serves...as a barometer of effort, as an indicator of stress, as a measure of health, and also as a literal lifesaver: If it weren't for sweat cooling our bodies down and flushing our toxins out, we'd all perish much sooner."[13]

Question: How important is your healthy sweat function; as induced by exercise, or rocking your bed, or activities of daily life?

Answer: Very important, when and if you choose to **thrive and strive**.

With these facts as charged context, let's proceed to our amazing energy and power systems. Bodily systems that you **tap** to party into your 90s.

What's the Best Way to Tap My Fiscal Account?

Having cash resources in your fiscal (with a F) account, you can tap them in these four time-sensitive ways.

1. The quickest method to withdraw money is to take it from your billfold or pocketbook. There are short-term limits to how many C-notes you can carry, right? *You **do** need to remember where you placed your billfold (and bifocals too).* Your first withdrawal method is quick, and it doesn't force you into debt. Yet it can only be tapped so often for so much.

2. The next expedient way to withdraw money is from an ATM machine. Withdrawals of your cached assets also have spending limits and need to be replenished before you can again tap the ATM.

3. The slowest, yet most enduring, method to tap stored savings is to continually visit your financial institution to make withdrawals from your "**utility**" account. This is a slow-twitch method to carry your nest egg well into

your fiscal future. Not inexhaustible, unless you are Bill Gates or Jeff Bezos or oracle of Omaha Warren Buffett, so think long-term.

4. A fourth (and contingent) way for resource withdrawals is to *again* visit your financial institution. If, and when, your **utility** account is low, you may need to take a valuable item from your security deposit box and sell it. There is, most assuredly, a price to pay for taking your withdrawals to this unusual limit.

There are also physical occasions when you may use a combination of these withdrawal techniques, right?

Once you have built capacious stores of energy in your body, you can physically (with a P) tap those reserves via four processes, in timed stages, just like your fiscal bank withdrawals (above).

1. The quickest withdrawal method is to convert energy already stored in your cells' tiny generating stations (called mitochondria). These withdrawals are convenient, fast, and effective, though these withdrawals cannot be done continuously. And they need to be replenished every few minutes. Cellular energy withdrawals are like your fiscal billfold or "Apple Pay."

2. The next way to tap your physical energy resources is to resupply those tiny powerhouses with potential energy already flowing in your bloodstream. This conversion of energy, which we call aerobic activity, is analogous to tapping your fiscal ATM. It too has withdrawal limits that can be exhausted. Think four grams of glucose flowing in your bloodstream – high potential, short lived – as in good for a few minutes' effort! *Luckily*, you have a physical overdraft protection system in reserve.

3. Our slowest yet most enduring method of resource withdrawal is to tap energy savings in our liver and/or from the storage vaults in our fat cells.

– There is *an unfortunate variation* to this withdrawal method. We might (regrettably) withdraw potential energy from muscles rather than liver glycogen or stored fat. That's a survival carryover still wired in our "reptilian" brain. Therefore, we try to avoid this ad hoc banking variation, right?

4. A fourth way to access our energy stores, when our aerobic bedrock method is depleting, is to "go anaerobic" and use an alternate energy source to sprint to our finish line, even after a long haul. This sprint method can tap short-lived, yet powerful potential of lactates in our circulatory system. Yet, there is a consequence of lactic acid buildup with cellular soreness after this withdrawal method is tapped.

Just as we cited for those four fiscal banking methods, we often use "combo" energy withdrawals for our physical work or play. This combo constitutes "overall" performance.

Repeat after me: There are *many times more calories* stored in fat than vaulted in our livers, blood system, or in our cells. Hence our innate endurance capacity to outlast by "fat burning." We humans perform better on "long" endurance runs than animals do because we can tap 9 calories of potential energy from each gram of storage fat. Right. The longer the distance, the better human runners perform vs.4-legged critters.

Yes, humans can run longer and faster than racehorses. Persistence and "bank-vaulted" aerobic capacity matter. Stored fat and aerobics helped our forebears catch dinner in Paleolithic days.

Baby, we're born to run long distances and to sweat. Remember, Springsteen is a KABOOMER.

Let's consider a thousand words in a picture for remaining details of STAMINA. Endurance to better move, breathe and sweat. To stayin' alive, longer and better.

Steps for Stamina—Your Key to Stayin' Alive

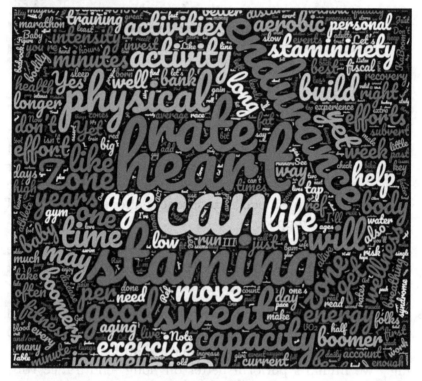

Repeat after Koach: I will breathe better, move more, and get sweaty. I may also recite poetry.

17 Words, 3 Lines

An endurance haiku from a Mayo Clinic physiologist, Michael Joyner, is worthy of your consideration:[14]

> *"Run a lot of miles,*
> *Some faster than your race pace,*
> *Rest, once in a while."*

Please *re-read* Joyner's poem, as it is *key* for your stamina and endurance. Volume matters more than pace. Recall our 80/20 baseline for time invested in heart rate (HR) zones. And do **not** forego rest.

A feel-good corollary to this poem is our innate capacity to reach our Second Wind.

Catch Your Second Wind

Pursue and experience *natural* opioid effects, which we commonly call our "second wind" or "runner's high." Your own runner's high is very special when you sustain aerobic effort long enough to sense those wonderful boosts without causing a problem with law enforcement. How long? It depends. Some folks can sense their intrinsic nirvanas after 45 minutes of aerobic activity. In my peak running days, I found my pretty consistent "highs" or uplifting second winds after about eight miles of footwork in 50 to 60 minutes. My legs feel lighter, striding seems effortless, and I'm high on life, sans morphine. Pretty special indeed. Go git yours!

Yes, sports other than running/jogging have their own stages of enlightenment. Run, swim, bike, hike, or row "a lot"— yet not too fast. This approach easily accommodates intense tennis, hustled pickle ball, or sets of volleyball as KABOOM-ER endurance activities. Golf? Probably not, unless you walk quickly and play fast for 18 to 36 holes. Note: Skipping heavy 19th hole libations or moderating your foursome's celebratory cocktails is probably wise.

Get your heart pumping and keep it pumping in a zone that you can sustain and in which you sweat. The mode of movement isn't as key as the motions you make. Not to get ahead of myself, but adequate hydration is important to sustain top performance in your sustained activities—whatever the weather.

You were born to move, sweat, and feel good—right? Remember Wolfman Jack!

When? Most days each week, most earthly days until your Doc raises a STOP sign.

Yes, sweat and party-time can and should be intertwined (unless you have a special physical or medical condition, that is). You pick the times of day, based on the activities of your daily life and your own biorhythms. Are sweating and weight loss related? You betcha.

Weight Loss?

Yes, you and I can lose weight from our endurance activities. Yet I assert that this intent is not a be-all and end-all reason for gaining stamina.

That "weight loss" factor is contingent on more than a few variables. Remember that you are unique. As a biochemical fact, a 42 kilometer jaunt (our modern marathon distance) for a male runner of "average" build burns one pound—that is correct—*about one pound of body fat* during the marathon. A half marathon run by that same male burns a half-pound of body fat (hopefully from the right energy source of fat rather than muscle). You *don't* really run a half or a full marathon with a priority to lose eight or 16 ounces of fat, *do you?* Post it! Unless endurance activity is complemented by strength activity, one may experience "skinny fatness," as our bodies may unfortunately consume muscle as an energy source. It's in our makeup.

Work *all* seven interrelated components of fitness and wellness to better your odds. Pounding the pavement, so to speak, is very good for ladies' bone densities, yet they (and their male counterparts) need resistance efforts too! KABOOM.

Growth and Repair

There are more important reasons to run, swim, or bike "long" distances (correlated to "long" exercise times) than just calorie burns. Consider your runner's highs, getting past the wall with your second wind, and tithing your bodily temple with sweat to trigger its restorative chemical processes.[15] Our processed chemical messengers – with profound anti-aging consequences – have arcane labels, so we'll skip them for now. You can contact your Koach, and/or attend a seminar to delve into the fascinating and arcane chemical messengers of restoration and growth.

Plus, endurance events stimulate healthy *brain* activity. Plus, a KABOOMER who trains for stamina should sleep better, if, one avoids over-training. A corollary is that one's increased circulation from aerobic exercise can increase libidinous performance. Do you recall the "DOA" finish line fate of Phidippides, the first marathon runner?

Low impact endurance activity, *unlike* Phidippides' double round-trip from Sparta to Athens in 490 BC, is great for nearly all. And mandatory if you're going to KABOOM. And I'll double down on the 80/20 low HR payoff.

Your WIFM Payoff as a KABOOMER (Redux)

Short answer: Your **Real** Gym Age is your *payoff*. (You don't need to belong to a gym to gauge your KABOOMER status). Here are non-gender numbers which **do** count.

- A KABOOMER is notably young in heart, mind and body. Younger in gym age than half of his or her age peers.

- Check my math...A top 10 percent KABOOMER is *younger* in gym years than 90 percent of all her or his age peers.

A very top KABOOMER is *younger* in gym years than 97 to 99 percent of **all** boomers. Here is a personal example for gym age vs. chronological age. An indoor rowing machine event— the 500-meter "sprint"—is long enough and hard enough to challenge anyone's sustained performance if he or she goes "red zone" for fastest completion time. According to *Men's Health* and other sources, one mark of a male's gym fitness and stamina, independent of age, is to complete a 500-meter row in under 90 seconds. Granted, I'm a pretty big KABOOMER guy. Yet I can complete this distance in under 90 seconds at my Medicare age, beating lots of younger and bigger dudes.

I've done quite well with my physical 401(k) account. And I can help you build yours.

I recommend a Men's Health gauge[16] of your fitness age to check on your "real" wellness and longevity factors. Lady KABOOMER, real gym age measures are different, yet just as important, for you. Please visit *wellpastforty.com* for women's gym age measures.

Is your "real" bodily age less than your chronological age? I hope so! And better yet, many of us can add years to our life by doing some simple yet hard things (like imbibing a wee bit less, and by managing our portions of clean nutrients).

Please, please try this Share Care application to gauge your "real age:" www.sharecare.com/static/realage.

When you do, you will see that endurance exercise and activity are key bodily factors. Yes, diet, stress, and genes are big factors in actuarial measures to live young(er). Yet, why not deal yourself a best possible hand, as Lodge and Crowley wrote, to be "**Younger Next Year**"?

I like to think that balladeer Bob Dylan was spot-on with his lyrics:

"But I was so much older, then. I'm younger than that now."

What's your inspiration to move more oxygen through your 60,000 miles of cardiovascular piping? Longevity, perhaps?

You see, cardiovascular "fitness" is credibly pegged by a calculation of your VO_2 max.[17,18] Hang on, these symbols are important! The V represents volume, and O_2 is bonded oxygen molecules. Betcha you know what the "max" means.

Whether or not you're blessed by nature with good lung plus "pump & pipe" capacity, your nurtured "pump" capacity is directly related to your prospect for longevity. Take note: KABOOMER aerobic capacities "substantially lower your risk of cardiovascular disease and premature death." I like this affordable "term insurance" with that funny name of VO_2 (as illustrated in four Tables below). Low risk sounds good to me!

Me?

My collegiate rowing coach invited Dr. Fritz Hagerman to measure our crew members' VO_2 maximum. My capacity to move oxygen helped move me into a racing crew! These many years later, I'll take my **VO_2** Max rating as a "gym age" **29**-year-old. Frankly, I worked to get that capacity on my KABOOM-ER journey. I enjoy outlasting "young whippersnappers" by working to sweat and by breathing. Do check your **VO_2** Max someday, because normal doctor visits won't assess this vital capacity.

These following four tables are invaluable prompts for stayin' alive. Two **VO_2** Max charts for age groups of women show statistical Risks for Heart Disease. And two for males who are keen on stayin' alive.

Take these profound and credible facts to your physical bank!

1. *Low* oxygen capacity –> **HIGH risk** for cardio problems.

2. *High* oxygen (VO2 Max) capacity -> **LOW risk** for heart issues.

Women's VO2 Max vs. chances for Cardiovascular Issues

Women's VO2 Max				
Rating /Age	20-29	30-39	40-49	50-59	60+
Superior	>41	>40	>36.9	>35.7	>31.4
Excellent	37-41	35.7-40	32.9-36.9	31.5-35.7	30.3-31.4
Good	33-36.9	31.5-35.6	29-32.8	27-31.4	24.5-30.2
Fair	29-32.9	27-31.4	24.5-28.9	22.8-26.9	20.2-24.4
Poor	23.6-28.9	22.8-26.9	21-24.4	20.2-22.7	17.5-20.1
Very Poor	<23.6	<22.8	<21	<20.2	<17.5

Rating /Age	20-39	40-49	50-59	60+
Top 20%	>41	>37.8	>33.6	>30.1
Middle 60%	28.8-40.9	26.7-37.7	23.6-33.5	20.4-30
Lowest 20%	<28.7	<26.6	<23.5	<20.3

VO2 Max and Cardiovascular Disease in Women

Highest risk of cardiovascular disease	Middle 60% (26% lower risk*)	Lowest health risk (37% less)

Men's VO2 MAX vs. chances for Cardiovascular Disease

Men's VO2 Max

Rating /Age	20-29	30-39	40-49	50-59	60+
Superior	>52.4	>49.4	>48	>45.3	>44.2
Excellent	46.5-52.4	45-49.4	43.8-48	41-45.3	36.5-44.2
Good	42.5-46.4	41-44.9	39-43.7	35.8-40.9	32.3-36.4
Fair	36.5-42.4	35.5-40.9	33.6-38.9	31-35.7	26.1-32.2
Poor	33-36.4	31.5-35.4	30.2-33.5	26.1-30.9	20.5-26
Very Poor	<33	<31.5	<30.2	<26.1	<20.5

Rating /Age	20-39	40-49	50-59	60+
Top 20%	>50.4	>47.3	>42	>37.8
Middle 60%	36.1-50.3	34.7-47.2	31.1-41.9	26.1-37.7
Lowest 20%	<36	<34.6	<31	<26

VO2 Max and Cardiovascular Disease in Men

Highest risk of cardiovascular disease	Middle 60% (18% lower risk*)	Lowest health risk (39% less)

Two *uber-critical* footnotes to these lively 2 by 2 Tables:

1. If you already have another health condition, like obesity or diabetes, improving your cardio fitness becomes even more critical!

2. Improving your cardio fitness by just 3.5 points (as improving from good to excellent on the charts), will lower your risk of premature death from any cause by 13 percent! You'd get similar health benefits by reducing your waist by 7 cm, or by lowering your blood pressure by 5 points."[19] Yes, you can live longer and better through motion and sweat! Are you Nordic?

Nordic Notes

A Norwegian tool estimates one's cardiovascular health. Just check Winter Olympic medal counts from that small Nordic country for relevance and for national health.

Make your six reasonably quick and easy entries at www.worldfitnesslevel.org/#/start in either "metric" height and weight or English units. Then view its generated guess of your current cardiovascular capacity (with strong implications for longevity and vitality).

Note: This capacity estimate is tuned to a global demographic of average adults. Thus, my measured VO₂ Max is higher than the estimation by this tool. Yet for most, this tool effectively baselines cardio *reward versus risk*.

Non-Nordic? Let's reinforce how some populations, like Seventh-day Adventists in Loma Linda, California, have bonus Blues for stayin' alive longer. Let's agree to agree that activities of daily life can extend life too.

Big Bonus Blues

I commend to you sustaining conclusions about **Blue Zone** centenarians, as authored by Dan Buettner.[20] These long-living (and happy) folks in select communities are not ul-tra-marathoners or uber-aerobic freaks of nature. Rather, their endurance activities tend to be those of regular daily life: walking, gardening, and moving amongst family members and friends. Hold that social thought for wellness and longevity.

We do *not* have to go *red zone* nutty, dwell at lactate threshold performances, do Badlands ultra-endurance events, or stretch toward the limits of human endurance. We should move, sweat, and breathe. And we should also eat, sleep, chill, get stronger, and stretch to subvert our "bell curve" aging process. The aging process for normal boomers is a scientific term that has lots of E's in it: *senescence*. It's a nice way of saying *deterioration* or *senility*. Sorry, but someone had to say it. Avoiding cellular senility (senescence) certainly appeals to me. Surprised?

Surprise!

Many of us recall what the book and movie character Forrest Gump shared about stamina: "I ran and ran...."

Forrest was indeed a KABOOMER! Gump's Momma offered timeless advice that "life is like a box of chocolates." She knew that surprises and unforeseen happenings await us all.

- You can't predict what you are going to get in your remaining days. Value your stamina as enduring capacity to help you face and overcome those surprise "gets."

Let me reiterate and reiterate: One very bitter chocolate which might be a surprise is **senescence**. A sad and life-threatening surprise *if* we are not prepared. Billions of our cells will ultimately get weary, hibernate, or shut down when their double helixes are damaged. Yes! And yes, we can **defer** and **delay** such intracellular damage.

How? Drumroll...*motion.* Motion is the bedrock of our physical 401(k)s, and it is supported by clean eating, and rest, and strength moves, and...

There is a big difference between *getting older* and *getting old.* Tailored aerobic exercise is widely accepted as key *"anti-aging"* medicine, regardless of chronological age, and exercise is **key** to our *"bioresilience.*[21] This is bodily resilience to offset alarming conditions of modern life. Such factors as poor-quality calories, limited activity, leaky gut, central obesity, and inflammation. These unhealthy conditions, these abnormalities, are grouped together as *"metabolic syndrome."*

If you play Jeopardy, ask the question for this category answer:

Alex Trebek: "An alarming condition or syndrome—without any known cures—which adversely affects one-third of all adults in America."

Question: What is **Metabolic Syndrome**?

Ding, ding as your just won Double for your smarts. Doctors and researchers at the Mayo Clinic define metabolic syndrome as:

"a cluster of conditions that occur together, increasing your risk of heart disease, stroke, and Type 2 Diabetes... increased blood pressure, high blood sugar, excess body fat around the waist, and abnormal cholesterol or triglyceride levels. Having just one of these conditions doesn't mean you have metabolic syndrome. But it does mean you have a greater risk of **serious disease**. And if you develop more of these conditions, your risk of complications, such as type 2 diabetes and heart disease, rises even higher."

"Serious disease?" You can do without that, I presume.

Did I hit you over the head with a big enough hammer? (Hammer Dave is a rowing hashtag for me.) Good. Now I'll swing again to reinforce stamina's bedrock role in *your* health and wellness.

> "Older people can benefit greatly from exercise, especially to reduce their risk for developing metabolic syndrome… exercise can be as effective as what is accomplished today with drugs…and results also confirm the value of exercise for managing multiple risk factors. Because so many older persons have or are at risk for metabolic syndrome, this study provides a very strong reason for individuals to increase their physical activity levels. They will reduce their fatness, and increase their fitness and leanness, while reducing their risk for heart disease and diabetes…."[22]

We can **KABOOM** our way to *reduce* heart disease, diabetes, high blood pressure, bad fatty acid levels, and those other clustered risk conditions. Now, take care to give yourself some Rest and Restoration (R&R) for youthful fountains.

R&R

Please remember that you are no longer 20-something. Your maximum heart rate is lower; your skeletal muscle mass is lessened; and your body's recovery capacity has taken a downward hockey stick turn since your roarin' twenties. Ultra-distance veteran and trainer David Glover reminds us that **age** *does matter:*

"Masters athletes need to take into [their] account that their body will *recover slower* than when they were younger. *More* rest will also help prevent overuse injuries. Ways to improve recovery as a masters' athlete are to:

- Include *more* easy weeks within your training plan.
- Take one day off training per week.
- Listen to your body and don't attempt to train through sharp pain or injuries.

- Reduce the time you are on your feet outside of training.
- Aim for better quality sleep and more sleep; and
- Consume protein immediately post-workout to aid muscle repair."[22]

Note: Post-workout **recovery** is *not* synonymous with doing *nothing*.

You might drink to this...*Men's Health* advises that there is little wrong with a R&R beer after a strenuous stamina workout. I'll drink to that (moderately). Dogfish Head Brewers assert that their SeaQuench™ Ale is good for exercise recovery. I'm okay with that, and so is The Daily Meal as reference for *proper* adult hydration.[23]

Fire or Ice?

Hot or cold (fire or ice) treatments applied after your strenuous exercise may speed recovery. An ice bath between closely scheduled endurance events in hot weather worked for me. *Your* experimentation is the best way to find what recovery means work best for you for specific conditions. If I was a finisher of a marathon in Antarctica, I'll bet you can guess whether I'd prefer fire over ice after crossing the frozen finish line.

H O H... I advocate hydration before, during, and after activities lasting an hour or more in any exercise conditions. I know that my body can *only* absorb so much plain water when bouncing along a marathon racecourse or half-century bike ride. Right we can only tolerate a quart per hour, or so. That said, some electrolyte drinks bother my constitution. GU™ and similar replenishments taken on the run tend to bother me too. Each to his or her own. Let the color and timing of your urination help you drink adequate fluids or abstain during and after "sweaty" events. Imbibe *before* you sense thirst!

Remember that one of the first reasons for your or my decreased athletic performance is <u>dehydration.</u>

Human Kinetics[24] states that endurance performance starts to degrade after 2 percent water loss (by body weight). Trust me – you lose water from sweat and exhalation quicker than you think! Dehydration can be a degrading factor in almost any workout temperature. It is just as important to drink fluids wisely in cold workouts as it is in hot humid ones. Monitor your body to avert dehydration and heat stress/stroke maladies. Be safe, always. Breaking fast?

Eating Before My Stamina Activity?

Yes. I know some capable master's athletes who prefer to run, cycle, or row in a fasted condition, but that isn't me. I like a little something in my system for a morning or mid-day endurance event or activity. And I do eat more-than-my-normal portions of complex carbs for two nights before a competition. I also go very easy on pre-race alcohol consumption. Before a distance event, I ritually eat a big helping of spinach. Researchers that I trust state that amino acids in this green "superfood" help with one's "vasodilation" and may support one's improved aerobic performance. According to the Nitric Oxide Center, endurance in some researched conditions and events may improve by *16 percent. Trust but verify...And be mindful of supplementation.*

This Center's **golden rule** for supplementation is stressed:

"It is important to keep in mind the golden rule of supplements: *they won't do the work for you.*"

Do the work! Like you, I often hear about classic or newfangled boosts for performance. An old-fashioned trick from Momma Gump, or your mom may have merit too. If you can tolerate beet juice to help boost your nitric oxide (chemical symbol NO) levels for stamina, good on ya. I can. Are there other natural "tricks to treat" KABOOMER stamina? You bet-cha.

Ergogenics and Other Natural "Tricks"

A baby aspirin "digested" before a long run or race may help your stamina.

I assert that modest amounts of coffee (as in 1-2 cups) help me perform without having to search for a porta-potty.

Perhaps it is a *placebo* effect and no endorsement is intended, but I mention that over-the-counter SportLegs™ tablets may help. I take them—per recommended times and dosages—before my big endurance events. I cannot say, with certainty, whether SportLegs give me a biophysical racer's edge. Yet they might. They're safe and they are cheap for this cheapskate. Strange yet true that placebos can improve performance!

Here's a newish factor of "supplemental" interest: Cannabis. Why? Our US society is accepting this plant-based supplement for varied "legal" uses. Marijuana or cannabis, or the non-buzzed alternative Cannabidiol (CBD for short) just might help some runners deal with their race anxiety. And some runners or other endurance boomers just might find that their exercise recovery is aided. As a retired military guy, defense contractor, and reasonably conservative cheapster, your old dog author cannot speak about marijuana or CBD from personal experience. Find your mix.

Variety Is a Spice of Stamina Life

You might consider cross-training to mix it up so that efforts don't become dreaded drudgery. I do.

Some don't and that is okay. Example: A shirtsleeve KABOOMER relative became a marathon runner. He jogged the same training route at the same speed month after month and year after year. His good deeds were apparently at the "right" heart rates to qualify for the Boston Marathon in his age group. To train, he strapped on his shoes, put on his reflective gear, and ran that same distance course six nights a week (when not competing). Folks like him may be mentally tougher than I am, or they are better wired for discipline to get past drudgery of execution, day after day, month after month jogging, biking, walking, or swimming the same roadways, trails, or swim lanes for the same distances. Personally, I love a *mix* in my stamina activities. Routine is good, to a point, in my reckoning. You should be your own judge and jury. Experiment. Journal. Share experiences with your old and new friends. What works for them? What variety works for you to keep exercise fun as you avert aging?

Sweat and heart rate are your stamina keys, not your obsessing over stick-to-it routines or choices of endurance activities.

Periodization

Should you be interested in competition, there are certain buildup "cycle" times called *periodizations*[25] to help you train and peak for an endurance event. Both volume and intensity of effort are factored into your or bespoke periodizations by trainers or coaches, or by me. Note this stamina fact: A competitor can truly peak to "personal records" or top endurance performances *only* twice a year. Twice.

More on Training Cycles

Yes, in those weeks and months prior to your big event, it is progressive heart rate and volume effort (plus *sleep*) that build your cardiovascular and cardiorespiratory capacity—and not the specific racing exercise you pursue—that matters. Build your aerobic base (as big money in your bank vault) and avoid ennui to help keep your fitness fun.

Koach? Following my semi-annual *peak performance* for endurance events, my *preparatory period* is about two–four months in duration; my *pre-competition* period is one–two months long; and my *taper* period can be a few weeks to one month before a next "major" endurance competition. Post-event, I take *at least* a R&R week off from my sport in transition to preparatory efforts for my subsequent serial pursuit.

I'm sure that you know, or will learn, that Personal Records (PRs) are relatively infrequent, and are age dependent. My case: I don't run a 5:20 mile now, though I did in college as a *Clydesdale*. (In fact, my doctors had me give up middle-distance and long-distance running at age 49, after I ruptured my L5-S1 disc.) More recently, and thankfully less severely, my worsening elbow region tendonitis led to prolonged physical therapy. I cross-trained to remain sane until I could row and pursue my "PRs" again. I digress, yet this serves as a reminder that you too will get a ding or two in your wellness and fitness journey.

Dings aside, my maximum heart rate lowers as I age. Skeletal muscle mass will too. These are inviolate physical laws for us (naturally-fueled) mortals. This universal truth is why we generally compete in master's athletic events with our age-group peers. I love racing faster than younger rowers in crew, but winner's podium appearances are still satisfying when I prevail against my age peers.

Speaking of big events, you may hear about feats of endurance, such as a young dude running 50 "fast" marathon distances in 50 weeks. Impressive, yes. Is such a young person's feat one that a vast majority of us Americans should/could pursue? No.

I've taken enough of your otherwise perfect day or evening, so let's wrap up our thoughts to subvert senescence.

Be active to continue your heroic journey longer. Our journey may or not include PRs. Yet your modest or immodest journey for health and wellness should be longer and better.

"We must not *underestimate* how important physical activity is for health—even **modest** amounts can add years to our life," stated I-Min Lee, M.D., Sc.D., professor of Medicine, Harvard Medical School (see the National Cancer Institute study cited previously). That's what we're doin'. KABOOM.

Attention, Go – Later and longer

When is it "too late" to embark on a wellness journey with stamina? Well, it truly depends. "Never" isn't the best answer. *Later* than most think they can start is a good response. In most cases, "I can't or won't" embark on this journey is *unacceptable* as a response to me as your Koach.

Authoritative studies suggest that venerable adults should move regularly if they can get out of a chair, or if they can push a wheelchair or walker. When that person gives up on movement, senescence has won his or her aging battle.

Please consult your doctor and then self-analyze your return on invested capital—or sustained earnings to move and subvert "normal" aging. Your pursued stamina goals could be low, medium, or high. A 75–80 something person who is advised by his/her doctor to get moving should likely pursue *low* stamina goals. Think of brisk walks as fitting activity to offset aging and for *stayin' alive.*

Their Zone 1 conversational activities can and should be completed on four to six days each week *totaling at least* 180 minutes per week (3 hours), every week of each year. That's an average of 26 minutes per day, and those average 26 minutes can be parsed into smaller segments. Right. Government studies suggest that *moderate* activity of one hundred and fifty minutes per week can make *notable* differences in wellness. Your Koach suggests a 'lil bit extra. Poor Richard (B.

Franklin) and I call this a low barrier to entry for stamina; getting oneself into the comfort zone to build capacity over time and effort. If your Doc gives the readiness "okay," shoot for 30 minutes *more* per week weekly (or **180 total minutes**) than our Government recommends for "average" adults.

"Do a 180" to KABOOM.

One More Time

Each of us is unique in baseline capacity and upward aspirations for KABOOMER stamina.

Do check your resting heart rate (RHR) to ensure that you are not:

1. Over-trained from an intensive Zone II or III workout in the prior day or days.
2. Dehydrated; or
3. Coming down with a cold.

What Shoes Fit?

Great exercises or prolonged activity do wonders for *each* of us. Each action-hero effort to sweat and glisten should be fun and fulfilling. Proper intensity heart-pumping, decay-countering, aerobic energy-tapping activities include:

- Open water crawls or relaxing laps of pool swimming.
- Biking in our great outdoors or spinning indoors.
- Cross-country skiing.
- Hiking or rucking.
- Kayaking.
- Standup paddling; or
- Rowing.

A first principle for cardio-vascular health? Here it is:

Commit to *lengthy and relatively slow heart rate activity in one or more types of exercise* – until our partying stops. By "until," I mean *90 years of age or older.* Yup.

It is the worthy process of getting your cardiovascular system, your ticker, arteries, capillaries and veins, your tennis-court sized oxygen transfer capacity in each of your lungs, **and** your brain working in stride. Working in *unison* to sweat, with your heart beating in the "proper" training zone. You are destined to move and sweat.

Nature or nurture?

Is a KABOOMER made or born? **Yes.** Granted, the best enabler to become an uber-endurance athlete is to choose uber-endurance athletes as your parents. *Ha.*

- How big a left ventricle did you receive from your gene pool?
- What size lungs do you have?
- Is there longevity (as measured by "some" study demographic) in your family tree?
- Are your family and you relatively free of diseases/conditions like diabetes or fat metabolism disorders that impact a person's stamina or endurance?

Be breath-taking! Lung capacity and how quickly a baby boomer can fully exhale are proven marks of predicted longevity. *Figure on a 90th* birthday party trick. You will be able to knock out those many candles. Do keep a timeless tiger in your bank as prospects for that party trick are much better.

Bear with me as I restate a key KABOOMER point: What's done is done. What can and will be done isn't! Your KABOOMER epoch may be 30+ years long. Why not make what can be done in your earthly timeframe: breath-taking, age-defying and fun? Why not thrive and strive (to a point)?

Too Much of a Good Thing Is *Not* Wonderful

My apologies to Mae West. Fact: There are diminishing returns of *extended* time versus effort for endurance gains. Too much of a good thing is **offset** by known takeaways for stress injuries and stress-induced inflammation. As my personal rule of thumb for my activity, capacity building on an indoor rower or rowing on the water diminishes after *90 minutes.* There is still capacity building after that timed activity, *but* I've got grandkids to chase and yard work to do. And, ultra-stamina events may be hazardous to one's health. Why? Bodily functions can shut down. Inflammation/oxidative free radicals can rise to unhealthy levels for such studs of extreme stamina. If a rare individual, like less than 0.0001 percent of Americans, wants to competitively run a 100-mile race from Death Valley to Mount Whitney's portal in summertime, or jog through the night in California's High Sierras, more power to him or her. And remember that we are not quite as spry as we once were for most extended activities. (Toby Keith's great country and western song, with the line *"I'm as good once as I ever was"* is a great mantra for *some* KABOOMER actions). Marathon-running or century cycle rides? Not so much.

Likewise, for an ultra-distance "tough mudder" lady named Amelia Boone who performed until she was delirious.[26] She is awesome, yet she isn't of KABOOMER age.

Likewise, for a true KABOOMER, Diana Nyad, who persevered to successfully swim (non-stop) from Cuba to Florida. Impressive, but her feat would not be an attractive endurance journey for *me.* To my local male and female friends who swam across the English Channel, and circum-swam Manhattan Island: Kudos!

Century runs, climbing Mount Everest (unless you're a Sherpa), or cycling the 2,000-mile Tour de France, do **not** equate to centenarian longevity. Ultra-lessons learned for a true stamina "outlier," Christopher Bergland, can be reviewed in his great read: *The Athlete's Way: Sweat and the Biology of Bliss.*[27]

Chris ran on a treadmill for 24 hours straight, because "it was there," and because he was driven to do it. He *doesn't* recommend his extreme bowel discomfort, or his near organ shutdown as experiences for *you*. Chris asserts, as do I, that *sweat* is the key. For most of us, that equates to a single daily activity or workout session, or multi-sessions of "80/20" aerobics at least 30 minutes...five to six days a week.

Just get a little sweaty—often, being aware of over-exertion because you're *well past forty*.

Speaking of under-40 Jocks

They (and we) lose both endurance and strength capacity at linear rates until around age 70. Then our physical performance degrades at non-linear annual rates. Strength and sprint performances degrade more notably than stamina after age 70. In my approach, I prefer to stockpile what I can in my stamina stores before I reach my 70s. I can't defy laws of nature, but like you, I challenge them, safely.

SAFETY!!!

I'll wager that you, like me, regrettably know or knew a friend who was badly injured, or sadly suffered a worse outcome from a bicycling accident. Watch out for the other guy or gal!

And watch out for your loved ones and for yourself. Facebook's executive and Lean In leader Sheryl Sandberg, lost her husband in a tragic treadmill accident.

As the *Hill Street Blues* Sarge, Phil Esterhaus, cautioned at daily roll calls: *"Let's be careful out there![28]"* Be nimble and be on the proverbial lookout for curbs, holes, and obstacles in low-light times of day. And check Addendum B for more Safety guidelines.

• Carry a signal device and call for help for any instance of injury or bodily threat. Dog bites do happen. Ankle sprains and flat bike tires do occur. Be careful out there.

Other *forewarned is forearmed* safety reminders are:

1. Be aware of *hyponatremia.*[29] Too much hydration can be deadly in isolated cases.
2. Hydrate, even in cold weather activity.
3. Wear proper attire to head over the river and through the woods.
4. "See something, say something."

Caution a fellow athlete if you sense their heat- or cold-related symptom(s) might cause them harm.

5. Be ready to reduce someone's pain or help to save a life. Knowledge and practice of first aid, and familiarity with the proper use of automatic external defibrillators (AEDs), is a *must* for certified personal trainers. And it's not a bad idea for *all* of us to be locked and loaded as "good Samaritans." Tweaking one of Major Murphy's Laws:

"Working out is cheap; your life isn't.[30]**"**

Physical Readiness

Though I chose running as an endurance activity to share these stamina hacks, similar steps pertain to other endurance activities like road cycling, swimming, vigorous walking, or hiking. *Please* contact a local certified personal trainer if you are a challenged athlete in adaptive sports. *Likewise, if* you experience a muscle, neuro-muscular, bone, or respiratory challenge, check with a pro to suggest modifications to normal stamina regimens. And, thinking of normal, as in body parts...

1. Know your body. Measure your bodily dimensions that count:

    a. Leg Length:[31] A difference of leg lengths greater than five millimeters (one quarter inch) can contribute to lower back pain. If you have a leg length difference of greater than nine millimeters, then you have ~six times greater likelihood of lower back pain.⸱

    b. Asymmetrical "wheels" don't necessarily mean eschewing endurance activities on foot.   Applied technology, like orthotic inserts, can help avert join problems if you aren't symmetrical in your gait. *Few of us are perfect.*

    c. Check for gait imbalance: *over*pronation (ankles roll inward) or excess ankle supination (outward ankle rolling) while moving can lead to knee and hip joint or back problems. (See youtu.be/3UwZPz0C_zg.) Orthotics can help most individuals with pronator and supinator issues so they can experience "the joy of running" or striding.

2. See a medical professional regularly who understands KABOOMERs and their athletic needs. Even if nothing bothers or hurts ya, we males shouldn't do "guy things" like skipping medical advice. Gents, please see your MDs regularly! Ladies, this is also meant for you, though I can't offer experiential evidence. It's *just* anti-aging and quality of life we're jawboning for your next 30 years or more.

3. Wear proper shoes and gear.

    a. Find a shoe model with heel box and toe cup that fit each of your feet. Not too snug and not too loose.

    b. Don't run in your shoes for "too long." Breakdown of shoe tread and/or arch support will occur at some point.

    c. If you run enough, you may experience black and blue toenails. Hot spots or blisters, too. A dab of Vaseline jelly can avert or minimize potential blister sites, and Vaseline can also mitigate rubbed nipples and chafed thighs.

    d. Compression leggings or calf socks? Yes or no. It is up to you for comfort and for observed or perceived placebo benefits. Comfort and support matter.

e. Run barefoot? Not this Clydesdale. Try shoeless jogs if your foot toughness and mechanics allow. After all, barefoot runners pursued, and caught, their dinner for millions of years.

f. Athletic supporters are a personal choice for guys. This master's jock doesn't wear 'em.

g. Regarding a jogging brassiere or sport bra: be comfortably supported, ladies.

4. Intestinal distress may happen for endurance athletes of any age, in most extended activities with impact. Remember Satchel Paige's advice and think about bowels bouncing with every stride of jogging or running. Go easy on the fiber and spicy foods you eat before sustained endurance activities. I know—fiber and selective spiciness are good for sustenance—just *not* before your hour to two-hour jog.

5. Pick "right" surfaces to avert joint issues.

If you run on a bodacious beach for natural beauty or swimsuit scenery, like lucky coastal joggers, pick flat sand rather than *angled* surfaces for your striding. Your knees and hips will thank you.

6. Do your very best to avoid shin splints and plantar fasciitis (a common inflamed heel tissue and pain on the soles of one's feet).

a. Chill your inflamed and distressed connective tissue if injured.

b. Don't push to the door of discomfort or your pain portal – please! Listen to your bodily feedback. Pain *is* feedback, so **listen** to it.

7. Don't allow episodic or evolving physical issues to become chronic. I can speak from experience in this

regard. I (unknowingly) allowed a rower's elbow condition to worsen until it impacted my sleep with severe finger tingling. Be in the know, and roll.

   a. Use different sized balls or objects to roll your feet, calves and legs. My own rolling kit includes golf, field hockey, baseball, and softball-sized balls to hit my tight trigger points, roll away soreness, and hopefully flatten muscular knots.

     Hint: read your KABOOMER chapter for the **Stretch**ing element of wellness for more details.

8. Decide on solitary or group workouts for your stamina gains. I advocate blending solo or "group" boot camp/ team/crew activities—as a hybrid approach just as I advocate mixed methods in other KABOOMER chapters. Group workouts **may** well add to one's longevity. Tennis is a fun, social, and moving activity! Recent reports suggest that most of us should "*love*" one of the best "team sports" for overall wellness. Pickleball is ascending as another "team" event which is good in many ways. Strength? Not so much. Yet stretching, stress-not, stability, and *social* elements are true benefits of these KABOOMER activities.

Try a few, love at least one activity, and move at your right intensity to sweat in each.

If you want help, or think that you may need an assist, find it.

Find a Certified Personal Trainer?

I'm in business as a Master Fitness Trainer, champion master's rower, and sports coach. That stated, I tell every client that I intend to put myself out of business with him or her. Each needs to fly solo someday. I can help clients establish good habits for their journey. The rest of the journey is up to each KABOOMER, like you. Sure, I'm a life preserver, yet I'm *not* ever-present.

If your fiscal situation permits, research, vet and then try, a professional trainer. Be sure to check for shared expectations. If finances or life don't allow the employment of a trainer, worry not. Like supplements, trainers *can't* do the work for you. Breathe, move, and sweat in your chosen activity/activities. Maybe you can find a workout buddy with similar goals.

Away You Go

You know, it is a bit funny what a baby boomer remembers, and what he or she forgets. I don't remember my boomer birth in 1953, although my sainted Mom did. I checked into this crazy world weighing 10 loaves of Wonder bread.

I don't recall what I got for my first Christmas gift, when there were only two of us chubby Frosties in our bungalow. (Five other chubbies came soon after.) And I don't recall when or where we went on our first outdoor picnic, in our old Willys Jeep.

Yet I do remember the first time I finished my 42K (marathon) under three hours. I also recall trials and tribulations to put "money in my stamina bank," expand mitochondria and capillaries in my system, to sustain a race pace. I do recall my first collegiate rowing cup win. And I do reflect on injuries and conditions that I overcame; a herniated disk, a broken toe, skin cancers, sleep apnea.

Nowadays, I stay on my KABOOMER journey with planned, habitual stamina activities as bedrock for every *quality* day that I can grab. One day, I will blow out those ninety candles, vigorously. And each day, I will monitor my heart rate, breathe, and sweat.

I hope that you will too. Enlarge your physical 401(k) so that partying past 90 is *your* breath-taking prospect.

CHAPTER 3

More Than Pumping Iron — Why Strength Matters

What's that? Scotsmen like Braveheart were strang in their tongues and travails. Whether strang or strong, that condition is what a KABOOMER **needs to be**. Do I say that being strong to move stuff matters? Yes! Here is why strength matters, no matter your present condition.

> "There is no medicine that provides as many physical and mental benefits as regular resistance exercise."[32]—W.L. Westcott, Resistance Training Is Medicine: Effects of Strength Training on Health.

Right. Moving stuff is marvelous medicine! (Thanks for grasping that strength training = resistance training = moving stuff across a distance.) Make strang deposits to your physical 401(k) account, even if facing a condition like diabetes or multiple sclerosis. Benefits? Who walks away from benefits that help her/him live longer and better? Who doesn't want the vigor to party past 90? Your strength matters. Together, we'll peg decent, good, or great launch points for your bespoke strength/resistance training. Yes, you can. Yes, you should.

Before we focus on facts, let's consider three notional peers (as decent, good, and great actors). Our triad serves as context for how properly planned and executed strength programs **will** benefit each for longer and healthier lives. Let's meet Decent Deb, Good Garett, and Great George.

1. Decent Deb

Deb is a youngish divorced Boomer, born in 1963. Deb is a successful senior manager with three young adults as her offspring. She is the first responder for an aging Mum with early onset dementia. She was never a competitive athlete in her younger days, and she has an apple-shaped body type (somatype), also known as an endomorph. She would love to wear "sleeveless near 60" tops with pride, for work and for play. And she would like a leaner bod for wearing swimsuits. She does walk, but at a slow pace per mile.

After prompts from a co-worker, Deb took a credible health age questionnaire at www.exrx.net/Calculators/HealthAge to estimate her remaining years on this planet. She then realized that 30 more years wasn't enough for her (based on the Social Security Administration's actuarial mortality for her at 85). She wants to be fitter and to be an active grandma or nana when that blessed time arrives.

2. Good Garrett

Garrett, who was born in 1954, is comfortably easing into Medicare-aged life. He is happily married to the first love of his life, with one adult daughter who is now engaged to a Wall Street financial advisor. His wife is a decade younger than he is. She, gorgeous Ginny, is in very good shape, and she would like Garrett to be in very good shape too! Garrett was a competitive swimmer in college, yet life happened to him. His blood pressure is high, for instance. He wants to get closer to his athletic performances of yesteryear, and to improve his activities of both daily and nightly life.

His current measured body fat is "normal" as a mesomorph who can lose weight, yet he can also put on holiday weight if he isn't careful. His last blood draw showed a low testosterone level as compared to his peers. His "pear shaped" body profile suggests that he is not carrying "too much" visceral fat in his midsection. Some of his younger male and female pals have cajoled Garrett into long and hilly recreational bike rides on weekends. Yet he doesn't have the endurance for long "century" rides or the power for hill ascents with them. He wants to lower his "gym age" to be able to do that. He also notices that others' handshakes are firmer than his.

Garrett belongs to a "big box" gym and is sorta committed to weight workouts. He proactively took that same health age questionnaire,[33] as did Decent Deb. His actuarial life expectancy is 89 years, so he just misses a desirable KABOOM-ER benchmark to party past 90. He has read that resistance training can help his chances, in addition to minor lifestyle changes, like forgoing that single malt nightcap on weeknights.

3. Great George

George is a leading-edge boomer by age, as he came into this zany world in 1947 (that same birth year as Dolly Parton whom we cited in our KABOOMER introduction). George is blessed to have an ectomorph body type with only a slight "gut," and body fat that is considered "athletic" for a dude of his age. He had three kids with his second wife, after a practice matrimony that didn't last. And he continues to consult for businesses to stay active. His wife, nicknamed Georgie, encourages him to keep on keepin' on, and she asks George to move heavy stuff when needed. Yet, he progresses toward "skinny fat" in his body profile as years mount. He is unable to heft his grandkids or heavy suitcases like he once did. He missed a KABOOMER "gym age" mark for strength that matters.

His parents died in their 70s; one from cardiovascular disease and the other from cancer. He has been a relatively fast master's runner for half and full marathon distances for many years, and his endurance is very good. However, he has occasional back pain and a tight posterior chain. George wants to offset his progressive loss of muscle (sarcopenia in wonky terms) and start to branch out into cross-trained athletic competitions.

Your Koach knows that you are not exactly a Deb, Garrett or George. Yet what can work for them can indeed work for your Strength Matters program. Trust me. Now, to some facts.

Dragnet's Detective Joe Friday might (or might not) have deadpanned, "Just the Facts, ma'am."[34] Let's scrutinize these Facts that Strength Matters.

1. Increase your bone density (which is particularly critical for lady boomers).
2. Delay/diminish the 3–8 percent loss of skeletal muscle per decade from which Billy and Betty Boomer suffer. (This will reverse aging factors!)
3. Increase your lean (vital) body mass.
4. Increase your resting metabolic rate (meaning higher non-exercise calorie burn!).
5. Reduce your fat weight!
6. Improve your physical performance.
7. Allow you to walk faster (a valid longevity factor).
8. Allow you to stay independent longer (and party on).
9. Increase your insulin sensitivity to improve blood glucose management.
10. Assist in pain management for arthritis and fibromyalgia.

Hey Koach, is this list of facts complete? No, it is not. You will read more factual benefits as you turn these Strength Matters pages. Trust me. Strength matters mightily! Let's learn more about how we reduce aging factors by pumping it up, perhaps with biceps curl exercises as part of strang regimens...

Hey Deb, Garrett, George, and hey you: **resistance exercise is imperative as you strive to KABOOM**. As Doctor

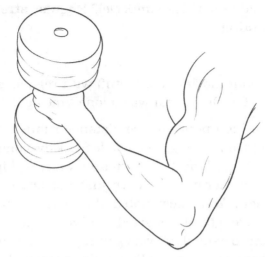

Dan Levitan recently wrote in Successful Aging, twelve men in the age range of Garrett, George (and me) significantly increased leg strength and muscle mass after just 3 months of strength training.

By this chapter's end, you'll have just the facts to sustain your KABOOMER Strength habits. You'll:

- Engage in properly planned resistance activities twice each week.
- Contract your muscles against loads in all three of your body planes (axes).
- Perform enough contractions to get a little bit sore and tight thereafter.
- Move stuff safely. Use proper form and loading. Consult medical and fitness professionals.

Why?

You do not want to lose flesh or weaken your bones! That is why.

KABOOMERs subvert sarcopenia by maintaining their skeletal muscles' mass and function. That terrible term sarcopenia has Greek roots: "sarx" or flesh + "penia" or loss.[35] Your best way to avoid loss of flesh (muscle)? **Regular strength or resistance training.**

Why Me?

I got serious about moving heavy stuff with regular strength training in my 30s. Okay, that was a long time ago....

Then, I was a high-performance distance runner. My running times were improving, yet my lean body composition wasn't. My measured neck-to-butt and waist-to-hip (WtH) ratios, even as a marathoner, were just not changing in a healthy direction. You likely noted that your metabolism, leanness, and strength also started to diminish just as your professional and personal life was getting hectic. Then those 40s came and went, and our silhouettes broadened and our youthful performances slipped more.

Please review what experts share about direct and indirect outcomes from sarcopenia! Think inflammation. Think cellular dysfunction. Think of adverse hormonal changes. Think of a sedentary life.

Now, shift to a higher gear. Activate your muscles and commit to strength habits that *subvert sarcopenia* and boost your metabolism. *Like medicine!* Don't look in your rear-view mirror of life, or fret about your current body composition, as that raises your *unhealthy* stress levels. Decent Deb doesn't need to be Jane Fonda. Good Garrett, likewise, you don't want or need to be Ahhhnold, but your competitive streak drives you to stay younger than your peers. Great George, you still can sustain athletic performance with proper regimens of resistance training. Look ahead to anticipate and act. Trust your Koach—*after* your medical doctor "sizes you up" and approves your liftin', pushin' and pullin'.

Does Size Matter?

Yes and No. Yes, size does matter, situationally. Bigger people can lift heavier (absolute) weights than smaller folks.

Why? They have more skeletal muscle around their bigger frames. Don't despair if you are not basketball-tall or linebacker-stout. Be proud of your KABOOMER kit, whatever it may be. Then get strong.

Example: Imagine that person A—let's call him or her Able Andy—has recruited and trained 45 percent of his/her muscle fibers to move objects. Let's call a second person Big Ben. Big Ben recruits just 30 percent of his fiber to move the same objects as Able Andy. Although Big Ben is larger in stature and has larger muscles, the smaller Able Andy may move heavy stuff in superior fashion. Your takeaway? You may, or may not, have big biceps. Yet KABOOMERs of most sizes and both genders gain *functional strength* to enhance their daily lives. And extend their lives. Make this note about recruited Functional Strength:

> *"Functional* strength training is going to *create healthy muscle growth.* When you reduce the fat on your body, you reduce your body's ability to store toxins; and when you combine that with an increase in muscle, you increase your metabolism and the ability to burn calories. Muscle is the **most** calorically active tissue of the body, so the more you have of it, the more calories you burn and the more you can eat. You also make yourself better at life's functional daily tasks. *There is no **skill** we call upon more in life than strength and the need for muscle."*[36]

Skills to grow muscle...reduce bodily storage of toxins... Increase metabolism...function better by day and night!

This next segment describes how one may be able to build muscular size and increase strength as your life skill. Take note that muscular size-building is a challenge for those of us at Medicare ages. It is more important to gain *functional strength.* To apply power effectively and safely for years to come. Dr. Westcott's seminal article, which was quoted earlier, documents "accumulating evidence that resistance exercise promotes muscle gains in men and women of <u>all</u> ages."[37] Note that universal adjective, all!

This good doctor didn't write that your resistance training regimen would be easy. He didn't cite a germane Olympic motto for stronger—Fortius— though he might have, as his message is to get stronger at any age.

Fortius

Doesn't *Fortius* sound solid? Like Fortitude. Like Fuerte. Think like an Olympian whose motto is "Citius, Altius, *Fortius*," meaning Faster, Higher, *Stronger*.

Strength was a matter of *life* and *death* in earlier eras. Legendary Spartans didn't become tough dudes without resistance training with muscular adaptation over time. Feats of strength were lauded in noble Olympic tradition, as they are to this day (and are now with women too). Let's overlook Olympian practices of naked "strongmen" in competition. Fast-forward to *strang* medieval Scottish highlanders like Braveheart, skipping what was or wasn't underneath their tartan kilts. Strongmen in those clans exhibited "heavy" skills in strength events like shot put, tug o' war, caber toss, and hammer throw. These were known as heavy events for good cause, and those brawny lads were revered for good cause. *Today's* KABOOMERs are revered by other boomers, kids, and grandkids, I assure you.

All strongmen and strongwomen invest in their robust physical 401(k) accounts. You can and should too. Themes of your healthy habits for *Strength Matters* are offered on the next page.

How as Homily

Move stuff repeatedly and you will get toned, stronger and more powerful. Enjoy habit-forming and life-saving repetitions by moving stuff twice a week, every week. With proper rest, diet, and stretching...

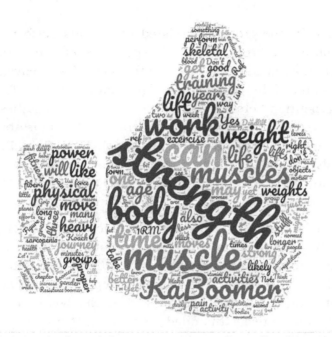

Yes! *Your bodyweight counts as good stuff.* I like to move it, move it and you should move it too. Seek other stuff too. Other objects do not need to be metallic weights or big box "weight machines." Resistance bands or Bodyblades™ or TRX™ suspension harnesses or sandbags. Or pushing and pulling a significant other. To grasp details of movement, our fitness community wants to be on good terms with you!

On Good Terms

Sequential moves without timeout are repetitive lifting, pulling, pushing, or twisting actions.

1. You lift, push, or pull "heavy" for absolute power in a few repetitions (one to six is deemed to be a few).
2. You lift "medium" weights to change your body composition and increase your muscle group sizes with more repetitions (eight to 12 counts of 'em).
3. You maintain muscular tone and sustain your acquired strength with more repetitions (15 or more) with relatively" light weights." Are you set to lift these three ways?

A "set" is one group of resisted repetitions performed before you take a break. There is a special repetition term—one repetition as maximum—that establishes what "heavy," "medium," and "light" objects or weights mean for you, for now. This repetition sets up your bespoke, timely activities on a leg or "period" of your strength journey. Get comfortable with these strength terms: **Repetitions(reps), 1RM, Sets, PB,** and **Periods.** It may take time to gain working knowledge of 'em. But you can't party all the time. The Power of 1 follows as your lead-off.

No, "1RM" isn't a rock group like Bachman Turner Overdrive. We use, and you'll become accustomed to using, this acronym to measure your strength actions with resistance equipment or objects. 1RM means **1 R**epetition of **M**aximum weight "worked" in one bodily lift or cycle. *WikiHow.Fitness* is quite instructive with added focus on 1RM matters of your strength.[37] Yes, a *protocol* to identify your current 1RM for a particular action (lift, pull, push, or twist) is a tad involved. Don't despair. Feel free to make a 411 call to a certified personal trainer to get your "max" or 1RM protocol right. 1RM Calculators (e.g., www.muscleforlife.com/one-rep-max-calculator/) are available as well. A key point is that *your 1RM should increase for each exercise (in about 8 weeks) as you advance* on your strength journey. Take that to the limit and consider rates of improvement:

- The biggest improvements likely occur *early* in your progressive strength journey.
- As you pursue 1RM upper "limits," your rate of increase for lifted, pushed, or pulled tonnage will likely decelerate. Just know and appreciate that your strength gains are non-linear. And be patient.

Another acronym you'll encounter is **"PB"** or **p**ersonal **b**est. (That "other" PB, peanut butter, is addressed as a healthy item for your sustenance in a later chapter. Healthy, that is, if you do not have peanut allergies.) Increases in your 1RMs *over time* and successive PBs *over time* are to be journaled and celebrated. Journal and celebrate as you stave off sarcopenia, rev up your metabolism, keep hormonal actions normal, and git it on. For completeness, you may hear "PR" as a shorter version of "**P**ersonal **R**ecord" in this context too. Consider PR and PB to be synonyms of strang merit. Make journal entries for either as you get KABOOMER strong. Period.

A *period* (or periodization) for resistance training is:

- Your established resistance routine to make progress until you reach a performance plateau (and you will).
- A strength or weightlifting periodization blends: 1. Volume; 2. Technique; and 3. Intensity. Enjoy this blend on a performance continuum, which are weeks to a few months long.

What Is Most Important for Your Very Own Matters of Strength?

Invest in your muscles and joints as much as you can—for as long as you can—to become the last one standing tall and partying at 90. This **is** an important investment, guaranteed.

Even if I've had a joint replacement? Yup! *Do not stop* moving/angling your original and bionic joints. Do your homework and avoid "some" movements that you might have done before your joint replacement.[38] See your medical doctor or health care professional. Listen to your body, your physical therapist, and possibly a professional trainer. You might start or resume your journey toward 90 candles with body weight moves, assisted progressions, and sets with limited ranges of motion. Did I mention that *motion is life for humans*? We are not sedentary plants; we are animals with behavior and locomotion.

So, let's start simply with our notional triad profiles of one boomer (Decent Deb) and two KABOOMERs, Garrett and

George, to shape your actionable resistance programs to become strang, then stay strang at almost any age.

1. Decent Deb

As you recall from our chapter lead-in, Deb is a boomer with body composition issues. Improvement areas like underarm bat wings and a muffin top waist, plus major mid-life stresses to bear. No wonder that restorative sleep is hard for her and comfort food became too accessible! Your Koach can help folks like Deb gain a general level of strength and fitness to change body composition and unhealthy fat levels. Better sleep and lower cortisol levels are likely, I assure you!

Deb wants and needs to achieve the median average of strength and fitness level of her *age and gender peers* in the general population. Can she perform work at about the same rate or activity measure(s) as her peers? This fundamental level of strength fitness means that she can carry on activities of daily life like her peers do. Hence, her notional descriptor of "decent."

Remember: the difference between ordinary and extraordinary is that little bit extra. A higher level of strength via those 'lil extras should appeal to you, and firmer arms and a smaller waist too! Let's add a little jest as zest, Deb:

> "Strength is the capacity to break a Hershey bar into four pieces with your bare hands and then eat just one of the pieces."—Judith Viorst, *Love & Guilt & The Meaning of Life, Etc.*

How appropriate willpower is for chocolate and for healthy habits! Deb, let's examine this journey one step at a time...

1. Call your doctor, please. Be cleared by your doctor to move objects.
2. Get a true baseline of how well you move your own body (weight).
   - Can you perform single leg lifts from a prone/face-up position?

- Are press-ups (a.k.a. pushups) from a face-down-on-floor position easy or hard?
- Can you climb steps two at a time?
- Can you walk a mile in under 16 minutes (a gym age marker for strength/longevity)?
- Can you get up from the ground without using your hands/arms—like you did as a young 'un?

If your answers today are "Nos", let's get you liftin', pushin' and pullin' stuff so that you can be stronger and leaner.

Strong Was, and Is, the New Skinny

Before Christ walked on water, a Greek Stoic named Seneca commended "simple exercises which tire the body rapidly... running, brandishing weights, and jumping."—*Seneca's Epistle 15[2]*[39] Sure, Seneca lived in male-dominant days, but brandishing weights will work for a stronger and skinnier you as well, Deb!

Strong women have *brandished* weights and charmed children of all ages. Fascination continues to current CrossFit games, plus World's Strongest Woman and Mrs. Muscles competitions. These impressive folks worked long and hard to gain their thicker and longer muscle fibers. You can't go back and pick stronger parents, but you can voluntarily work to thicken your skeletal muscles; regardless of your gene pool.

Lean forward, Deb. Consider a 19th century vaudeville performer, called Mrs. Hercules. Girl, she could brandish! I offer that impressive lady as an exemplar of strength matters and weights don't wait, because Strong **is** the new Skinny for you.

Deb, keep your willpower and sense of humor, like Judith Viorst mentioned, as you power through your strength session (with others, or with my assistance if needed). I nominate Ms. Viorst to be an honorary KABOOMER, by the way.

Figure out what reasonable weights or loads you should begin with. Or consult a knowledgeable cohort. Or find a certified personal trainer who fits with your attitude and goals. You are the client, after all. I recommend two dailyburn. com strength hacks that will help you to get started "without looking like a total newbie."

1. "Come into the gym with a plan."
2. "Pick the right weights."

(*I also recommend this daily burn link: Strength Training Tips for the Body You Want.*[40])

Start simple, Deb. Proceed slowly and learn as you go!

Strength movements for single muscles or muscle groups are fine as starters. These are generally called "isolation" lifts. Many gym machines are designed for your isolation lifts. And don't get psyched out by loud huffing and puffing by young guys at the gym. Just zone into what *you* need to do.

A biceps curl set with your purchased 5-lb. bag of sugar is fine for your early resistance exercise. No gym costs or space are required. Likewise, for a bodyweight pushup, as this KA-BOOMER couple is performing here:

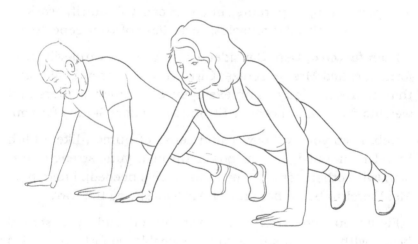

Deb: Think *long*. You need to perform long and slow routines to change your body composition over a few months' time. (Note: Further along your journey, you can periodically "tone" your thicker and longer muscles with higher repetitions of 15 or more with lighter weights per each set.)

Meanwhile, lift or move with eight to 12 repetitions of heavy enough stuff. In three sets. That is 24 to 36 total movements of your exercise with the right weight (resistance).

Loading is your key to impact those flabby arms and waist. A rule of thumb for proper "loading" is this: If you can perform more than *12* repetitions of a given weight routine in a "set," your weight is too light to change your body composition. With that dozen or more reps, you are focused on endured strength and muscle toning. Not bad in any way, yet those higher reps/lighter weights aren't prime for changing to swimsuit readiness.

Deb, you can and should take these words of periodization pros at BreakingFitness.com to your bank: "If you have been training consistently for less than two years, you are a **beginner in training age.** Add five pounds for upper body movements or ten pounds for lower body movements every training session in a progressive fashion until you plateau. Then reset and begin again."

Deb:

1. You may be a disciplined self-starter. If so, YouTube and Dr. Google may suffice for freebie resources to improve your body composition. And Verywell.com is a fine resource of daily informational tidbits if you are interested, and I trust that you are.
2. Or you may want/need a helping hand to enable your journey past the beginner stage. If you can afford a certified personal trainer, go for it. Note: Cookie cutter strength plans are verboten. You need a bespoke strength program that is designed, and that will work,

for you! Do not allow a trainer or coach to offer you a cookie-cutter or a young person periodization.

3. Or, if you're lucky enough to have a learned pal to be your strength workout buddy – yippee!

Whichever... START and sustain efforts for weights that don't WAIT.

And, very importantly, please know that your good results take time. Plan for six to eight weeks of weight training and moving stuff before you feel, sense, and see the results of your physical and mental investment. You will see a difference when you don your clothes, and a "delta" in your evolving feats of strength. This timed improvement benchmark is based on twice-weekly sessions of "hypertrophy"[41] to change your body composition. It must also be based on YOU.

We KABOOMERs benefit from **two** rest days before working those same muscle groups again. Hence, work your *twice-weekly strength plan* rather than the thrice-weekly plans which are built for younger athletes.

Yes, you can alternate muscle group days to lift on more days each week. My personal preference is to do my whole-body resistance (strength) training twice each week with two days of rest between my "work." I hit all major muscle groups in each one. Monday/Thursday or Tuesday/Friday or Wednesday/Sunday pairs are my strength sessions each week.

Also, please take a day off each week, with stretching and low intensity cardio-activity for your strength and stamina Sabbath. There is a reason why we Americans call our Sundays "days of rest," right?

I include whole or total bodywork in all three of our body planes in most of my strength workouts. (Remember: front-to-back, side-to-side, and twisting body planes). Now for one more necessary four-letter acronym: DOMS.

DOMS: Not Sore, no Score.

Delayed **O**nset of **M**uscle **S**oreness (DOMS) *will* greet you, Deb, after a proper strength workout. In my strength journey to suppress sarcopenia, I'm sore the next day; then quite sore on my second day after serious strength workouts. I suspect that you will be too. That second day soreness and tightness "comes with the **trophy** territory."

Hypertrophy stems from the Greek roots of "excess" and "nourishment." I like the sound of those *growing* roots, and I appreciate growth. Deb, please take note of this key: you need to work those muscles to cause "micro-tears" in them before they can get bigger and longer. And "gym age" trophies *are* within your grasp.

How do you grow, Koach?

Great query. Just remember that I am different from each, and every KABOOMER. And remember that I am not always pursuing muscle growth. There are periods each year when I focus on *power* (3-6 reps with heavy weights) or on *endurance/toning* (15 reps or more with light weights). You should also vary your strength work regimens. And vary your hand grips and foot stances too – for steppin' spiciness.

a. I deadlift, squat, and lunge for my lower body (baseline) work.
b. I do pull-ups, bench presses, and bent rows for my main upper body lifts.
c. I will perform one complex move that uses many muscle groups and hits two body planes. An example is a 'lunge, curl, press, twist' series move. Try it, you'll likely like it.
d. I also add a few *focused* exercises, such as a triceps series, or stability moves like pistol squats or single leg deadlifts with light weights. Please visit wellpastforty. com/resources for images and videos of strength moves/ variations. *Deb, as an example, you need a tuned triceps series to work those upper arms!*

In toto, I generally lift 8-12 times in slow repetitions across three sets. That is 24-36 total repetitions with good form. With slow negative (eccentric) phase movements that build. Deb's *standard lifts (steps a-d above) take about 45 minutes of weight work—twice a week to change her body.*

I add a few minutes of dynamic stretching before this workout. Then a cool-down with foam roller work (with the fancy name of self-myofascial release or SMR). Add longer static stretches to tally about two total hours a week. Right-O. About two hours of weekly weights to add years to your life and life to your years. KABOOM, Deb.

I ask your pardon that I omit many wonderful weighty moves without stepped explanations. As **KABOOMER: Thriving and Striving into your 90s** is page limited, please circle back to me, or visit the Well Past Forty websites to gain specifics for your proper form of **E**xercise that beats **D**rugs.

Note: Like Deb, some of you may need a lifeline regarding proper starting form and movements. Take your time and invest your effort to get these strength moves right. These are the cornerstone moves for your physical 401(k) account.

Safely move stuff at times that work for you. Get your rest days. And replenish your muscles with healthy nutrients plus water.

Was that yet another linkage reminder? You bet, as strength and sustenance elements strongly intersect. Eat healthy and nutritious foods. Reduce your caloric intake as needed if body fat or mass is an issue. But do **not** diet *without* resistance exercise as a companion. Remember that increased muscle increases your resting metabolism for calorie loss and decreases your fat levels over time. Don't wait until you are skinny fat.

How about folks beyond that beginner stage for weight work, where Decent Deb currently finds herself? Let's gain from Good Garrett's story as a strength practitioner.

2. Good Garrett

Garrett, well done! Your profile sounds like you apply your time and talent in your journey to become stronger and fitter than about three-quarters (75 percent) of your age and gender peers. This is excellent strength, as you're in the top quartile of all your age peers, a card-carrying, bell ringin' KA-BOOMER.

My strength triad for Deb, Garrett and George as representatives doesn't conform to "normal" population bell curve. It is not intended to be normal. It isn't about normal strength and applied power versus a general population of 75 million other Americans. It is about you, Garrett, living better and longer because you have forced your body to "voluntarily" adapt to resistance loads you placed on it. Why wither from loss of flesh?

Tellin' You Why

Seneca and his quiet toga-clad colleagues were onto something that you should take to the bank, Garrett. Consider your *brandished* strength as a natural shining way to counter mind fog, dementia, and worse things that could be happening to our noggins and bodies. And to keep your young and fit wife content. And please remember that key modifier "*simple.*" Another two tremendous merits:

1. Manage type 2 diabetes and blood sugar levels, if you are so afflicted.
2. Improve cardiac health and avoid strokes.

Adding merit badges, I offer even more valid reasons for you to lift weights:

1. Lower *unhealthy* abdominal fat.
2. Reduce cancer risk.
3. Lower injury risk.
4. Strengthen mental health and resilience.

5. Improve flexibility and mobility. (Wait for "strengthen to lengthen" efforts in your future chapter.)
6. Enhance your body image and composition.[42]

As Hans and Franz used to say on Saturday Night Live: "Pump You Up" (I add "naturally"). Ready for your natural Pump or Boost? Now that you are ready, you should anticipate an occasional ache or pain. Garrett, as a first step (after your regular MD checkup, that is), mold your mighty grip please.

Get a Grip

You might like old-time strength moves described by G. Jowett (1932) for "Molding a Mighty Grip." Did I have a special reason for mentioning mighty grips? Yes, I did.

Your **grip** strength, which is easily tested with a hand-held dynamometer, is a validated measure of longevity. Yes, sir. Yes, ma'am. *A strong grip = a likely longer life with vigor.* You should make **grip** deposits to your physical bank account regularly. I offer two compelling reasons to get vice grips:

"Muscle weakness, defined as a grip-strength measurement of less than 26 kilograms (57 pounds) for men, and less than 16 kg (35 pounds) for women, was associated with higher overall risk of death and higher risk for specific illnesses."

"People with the lowest grip strengths ... were more likely to smoke, to be obese and to have higher waist circumference and body fat percentage. They also ate fewer fruits and vegetables, exercised less, and watched TV more."[43] See why you need a **grip**?

Rowers like me develop strong grips. I don't bend silver dollars, but I can grip a dynamometer and apply about 150 pounds of pressure with either hand.

You, Garrett, must **get a grip**.

Garrett, if you already have your strength workout and activity session planned and established then raise your bar with this 3-stage workout protocol:

- Lift,
- Record it, and
- Adapt your load as necessary.

Yours is a calculated journey to move stuff enough to elevate your heart rate and grow your muscle fibers over time. To intentionally cause "micro-tears" in your skeletal muscles from their contractions and extensions. Yes, you self-inflict little tears in your muscle fibers, which then thicken and lengthen after their rest and recovery time. Tear down a bit first in order to build up.

Hey Koach, does proper *form* matter? Great query, Garrett. Yes indeed.

What should I check after a set of strength moves or weight lift repetitions?

Check your exercised and elevated heart rate (HR). Is that rate in the right training zone? Are you breathing harder? Are you sweating? Are your exercised muscles tired or fatigued? If you answered "yes" to these checks, then you likely "did the work" to improve your strength. And you'll likely sleep better, unless you overdid the volume or intensity of your periodized routine.

Question: What is compelling proof of your strength efforts/ progress? Answer: If you're a 'lil bit sore and tight on any day that ends in a "y", you are progressing toward STRANG or FORTIUS!

Garrett, there are as many recommendations for strength training programs as there are pills in Carter's pill boxes. For example, the *Art of Manliness* website offers well-documented strength-training programs. Though this link says manliness, women too should engage in resistance programs, which are truly gender neutral, as you'll see. If a woman want to check a website "specifically for spitfires of your gender," try spitfireathlete.com.

We *won't* let your eyes glaze with too much information or "TMI" for details of a perfect weightlifting/strength regimen or progression. However, comma...

1. Challenge your biggest muscle groups—your glutes, quads, and lats - with prescribed lifting sets and with proper loading.
2. Progress with more/complex strength movements that challenge multiple muscle groups. These are great for your calorie burn so that you can have seconds of Ginny's gourmet meals without guilt or weight gain. You'll soon read about these multiple muscle group, "whole body" exercises, such as the "king" or "queen" of resistance lifts—the Deadweight lift or Deadlift.
3. Execute with whole body movements that take place in multiple body planes of motion.

Progress through stable strength and power moves in your strength program. Then, when that is established, start to work unilateral and "unstable" moves that combine strength and stability. Think of a single leg deadlift, and a compound lunge push and twist move as examples of "unstable" moves that you should tackle, for sure, when ready.

First, move stuff (or your body) with your isolated muscle groups. Second, progress to stable, complex moves that challenge many of your muscle groups. And when you are ready, move progressively heavy stuff in asymmetrical ways or from unstable starting points. I'm not speaking of tipsy sailor instability. You should ultimately move stuff, like you did as a kid, on one leg. Or on an inflated workout ball.

Feel free to research "lift" protocols on your own, or work with a certified personal trainer to learn, then perform, vital strength routines. Find what works best for you. Repeat after Koach: **This is medicine**!

In a galaxy far, far away, a Jedi knight once offered: "Use the force, Luke."—George Lucas, Star Wars

Use your newfound "medicinal" force and strength to put younger hill cyclists in your rearview mirror, Garrett! You should lift long, like Decent Deb is now doing, to KABOOM. And add heavy to your routine for explosive strength.

Heavy. Choose heavy weights with which you can perform (at most) six "good form and speed" repetitions in a set, per movement. Then you are lifting heavy for generated human power. Heavy is good. Remember Seneca's brandished word. Recall Dr. Westcott's medicine.

There is no heavier lift example than the eponymous Dead-weight Lift[44]—honest! So here is your heavy protocol.

Deadlifting Protocol

Proper Deadlifts are "mass builders." Think of mass in relative terms. In our third act of life, we just can't get bulked up or "mass-y" without the use of unnatural supplements. So make your muscle fiber chain to deadlift a 'lil bit thicker and longer. KABOOM safely.

- Proper form is very important when you're moving heavy stuff.
- Safety first is a deadlift imperative.
- Use a spotter.

We can *deadlift* heavier weights than in any other strength move. Note this benchmark: A beginner weightlifter, in generally good shape, should deadlift a 1RM which is **three-fourths** of her or his body weight. That is a *guideline*, so *don't be too concerned if you are "not there yet." Just get hands-on & lift.*

We also load our connective tissue, skeleton, and cardiovascular systems mightily in this lift. By using most of our body's major muscle groups in deadlifts, we can: 1. build mass (in the right hypertrophy protocol); 2. generate amazing power as a *1RM* "Olympic" lift; or 3. sustain complex repetitions of whole-body deadlifts versus time. Yes, focused variations of this King (*not Elvis*) and Queen of weight lifts abound. Try them, like this lady KABOOMER below:

Deadlift with Barbell—Posterior View

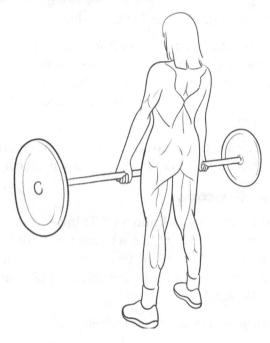

Shock or Awe? As a performance marker, recent USA Powerlifting records in 60-year-old categories for Deadlifts are:

- Women: 248 pounds for a woman weighing 148 pounds.
- Men: 435 pounds for a guy weighing 132 pounds. Yup.

What about your Koach? My master's rowing benchmark for deadlifts is 2.0 times my current body weight. That's 415-420 pounds. As weightlifting works, this means that I should perform 70 percent of my "1RM" ten times in a set *if* hypertrophy is my periodic goal. That's 288 pounds in 10 repetitions per set. And I perform three sets for those hypertrophy gains.

I use lighter weights when I adjust to lift *long* in my periodizations. I use heavier weights on the barbell if I am powerlifting them (in fewer repetitions of 1-6 per set). Remember variety for your strength moves.

The <u>same</u> "lift factor" as mine pertains to master's women rowers. Strong? Yes indeed.

- Primary "agonist" muscles used to Deadlift are your: gluteus maximus, gluteus medius (middle and posterior fibers), and hamstrings. Did I mention that the three gluteal muscles that combine to shape your buns are a **most powerful** muscle group in your boomer body (that is, if you do not sit excessively and/or acquire "gluteal amnesia" aka "dormant butt")?
- Secondary muscles used to Deadlift are your erector spinae, latissimus dorsi, and wrist flexors.
- Many other muscle groups are *antagonistic* supporters of your deadlifts. Garrett, grasp that stuff and safely contract those major muscle groups via repetition rates and ranges as prescribed by experts.

Certified personal trainers, and Master Fitness Trainers like me, follow the formal guidance of our certifying organization(s) for proper form. Check www.nfpt.com/blog/importance-proper-form-strength-training for a thorough checklist and protocol, with safety, and range of motion for deadlifting.

My MFT certifying body, the National Federation of Professional Trainers (NFPT), also offers excellent deadlift guidance.[45] Guidance for phases, form, and mistakes that lifters can make, in this great exercise for "everyone from athletes to the general population." BarBend.com is one site that you may have already visited. Another resource for proper deadlifting is: stronglifts.com/deadlift. I didn't say *improper...*

Avoid seven common Deadlift mistakes:

1. Duh—too much weight

2. Double duh—bad form
3. Pelvic tilting
4. Shrugging shoulders
5. Rounding your back *(Check your form in a mirror and/ or ask your spotter or certified personal trainer for his or her feedback)*
6. Knees caving toward the midline of your body
7. Rising up on your toes.

Wanna be a sumo deadlifter? I do and I am one; when I use narrower hand grips and wide out-pointed feet to position these deadlifts. Sumo Deadlifts offer shifts of emphasis on your exercised muscle groups.

Incidentally, sumo leg positions also work for another amazing lift—the **Squat**. That is prompt to call your Koach, Garrett, for squat protocols.... To whet your appetite, a male back-squatter is shown in good form below (with heels down, core tight, barbell resting wide on muscle rather than bone, with a fairly straight back).

Male KABOOMER Back Squatting

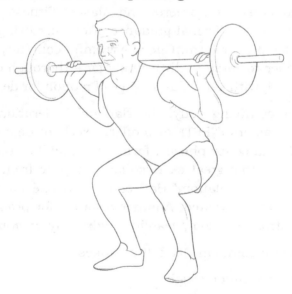

Garrett, you've become stronger and fitter than about three-quarters of your age and gender peers. This is *pretty good* strength.

Should you have your eye on a prize in your strength journey, you can climb to our Fortius victory stand, and meet Great George there. Anything else on your mind? Ahhh, ergogenics and supplements for muscle.

Are supplements safe? No and yes. Scientists have a name for natural boosts—*ergogenics*—in contrast to synthetic boosts for our physical performance. It seems ironic that a Russian medical source[46] defines ergogenic as a drug that "eliminates fatigue symptoms." Here are your Koach's takes on a few natural supplements that might reduce fatigue.

- *Coffee and tea* are broadly considered to be safe and wellness-promoting ergogenics. That is a conditional **yes**.
- *Nicotine*? Even though it is a natural plant compound, not so much, in my opinion.
- *Steroids or 'roids*? Inject or ingest synthetic substitutes for our strength hormones? **No**. Steroids are *no* laughing matter. And "badassness" isn't a laughing matter either when Chuck Norris walks into a bar.... (P.S. Badass Chuck Norris was born in 1940, so we can't claim him as a KABOOMER peer.) A ghastly snapshot of side effects caused by "whatever it takes" steroids is offered by our National Institute of Health.[47] *Au naturel* is the way to go. Be a natural badass with weights as your business. Embrace fatigue naturally. Fatigue is positive feedback that your efforts to move stuff are working!
- *Pump it up with testosterone and growth hormone?* Nope, unless your medical professional subscribes those supplements for true health reasons. Rather, I advocate exercise and diet methods to naturally boost "T" for both men and women. Yes sir. Yes ma'am.

- *Creatine, L-Citrulline, L-Carnitine, and Branched-Chain Amino Acids (BCAA)?* Maybe. Our Food and Drug Administration (FDA) does not regulate ergogenics, like these "performance" compounds, which our bodies naturally made more of when we were younger. According to the FDA, "Safety issues of long-term use, however, have not been addressed satisfactorily."[48] Now, do I use any of these "natural" ergogenics? Yes. In my sample size of one, L-Citrulline does increase blood flow via crafty chemical conversions for Nitric Oxide (symbol NO). This "NO" is good; trust me.

Please **don't** take synthetic shortcuts on your journey to vigor and brandishing weights.

Let's next work on Great George's strength plan as a **top five percent** KABOOMER.

3. Great George

Even though you run relatively fast on "long" flatland courses, George, you may be in extremis for your key strength parameter. That's true—approaching extremis—for becoming a 70-something, bent-over, shrunken guy, like actor Artie Johnson on Laugh In. And your wife, Georgie, hopes you can work on your flagging libido.

Wouldn't you rather jog uphill with pumping arms and beefier quads as a vital KABOOMER? Contemplate this stalwart statement from J.R.R. Tolkien:

"The oak that is strong does not wither."

What does *Lord of the Rings* mean by *wither*? Here is what: one's elder flesh and sinew can wither if he or she allow it. Tolkien didn't call that withering "sarcopenia." But medical doctors do. "*Sarcopenia* is...progressive and generalized loss of skeletal muscle mass and strength, and it is *strictly correlated* with physical disability, poor quality of life, and death."[49]

George, did you actively read that quote? *Disability, poor quality of life, and death*! I won't stand for it, and neither should you. Rather, beat sarcopenia. Experts say your secret sauce to beat it is...drumroll, Ringo...

Resistance work! What objects could you use as resistance? How about the remote control resting with you on your comfortable couch, along with that bag of Cheetos? No. Those unhealthy couch potato items won't offset or negate a withering of muscle. Be an oak rather than a sapling.

Resistance work against "loads" is essential for you to *stand tall, avoid a fall, and be the envy of all*. Let Brad and Betty Boomer envy you. And Decent Deb. And Garrett, too. Perhaps you'll inspire them to become strong KABOOMERs too. And you can power your way up tougher hilly courses with improved strength. And do not neglect the desires of Georgie.

Why Weights Can't Wait

George, these objects are your true cornerstone solution "as medicine." Let's reboot on your physical banking...First, recall that stamina is the bedrock of your KABOOMER life. Know that your restful sleep is the capstone of your physical 401(k). Now, strength is your cornerstone; that foundational stone of your bank of physical capacity to live long and well. Your strength for un-withering human fitness. Being strang like Scottish highlanders is to thrive and strive. Here is **strength** defined:

one's applied force and resistance against his or her muscular contractions.

What Captain America or The Hulk moves isn't worth a hoot to you, George. Or to me either. Being strong as an ox isn't worth a hoot. *What* **you** *move and how often you move it is certainly* a hoot. *And that is priceless.*

Move heavy-enough objects twice a week, every week, to achieve *stamininety*. This is achieved with two types of resistance moves, labeled isotonic and isometric efforts.

1. Our "primary" type of strength training is *isotonic*, because our skeletal joints move with **muscular contractions**.

2. A second type of strength activity is *isometric*, in which contractions occur, yet our joints are immobile. You might think of sumo wrestlers leaning on each other in stationary fashion as isometrics. Here is an isometric arm exercise:

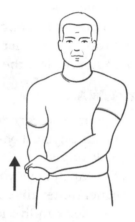

George, your Koach *isn't* discounting isometric work. I use isometrics when I'm trapped in coach class airline seats. And I **plank** often when I'm on terra firma. And I wall sit (See a Figure in our "Accident Insurance" chapter). And I hold the prisoner squat position with my *glutes to ground*. Some rhyme that isometric pose as a a$%-to-grass squat, yet I like "glutes to ground" better. (My Mum would *wash my mouth out with soap if* I was caught saying a$%.) And I do stationary yoga asanas, like tree poses. You should too! Take note.

Embrace *both* **isometric** (joint-moving) and isometric (joints-fixed) strength activities to KABOOM.

Bear with me for 2 technical sets for isotonic muscle movement.

- "Equal tension" phases of isotonic muscular contractions are: 1. concentric and 2. eccentric.

- Muscle groups generally serve as either a) agonists or b) antagonists in your isotonic strength moves. You'll learn more about these four terms. Just note 'em for now. Weights *can't* wait, but these definitions can. And speaking of your contractions...

Contractions, Chemicals, and Change

George, here is how your skeletal muscles gain size and strength to stand tall and wither not.

1. Your central nervous system stimulates your skeletal muscles to contract.
2. Motion occurs, and work gets done as your muscle fibers chemically expend energy (while "burning" calories).

   a. And muscles metabolize calories more than non-vital tissues in our body. More muscle equals more calories burned at work or play, by night or day.

3. Chemical messengers in our bodies are triggered as our muscles experience micro-injury with inflammation after their work. (Muscle repair and recovery is then completed in a day or two, depending on your age and personal factors. Hence your Koach recommends two recovery days between strength efforts for the same muscle group(s)).

4. Your work-adapted muscles become a tiny bit thicker and longer after "right" movements against resistance. Over 6 to 8 weeks, those tiny changes become noticeable. (Though humble, you are allowed to like kudos you earned!)

5. You improve your capacity to apply a bit more force in your next period or cycle of lifting, pushing or pulling stuff. KABOOM.

*__Note:__ Skeletal muscles are our voluntary tissues that control every action we consciously perform. Most skeletal muscles are attached to two bones across a joint, so these muscles move parts of those bones closer to each other in their (isotonic) contractions. In short, skeletal muscles support and hold up our skeleton. Skeletal muscles make us mobile—past 90 years of age—after one's **Weights don't Wait** habits are formed and kept. Feel stronger?

"What doesn't kill us makes us stronger."—Friedrich Nietzsche

Pay your price of admission, George, to get strang and stay that way.

Prices Paid

Your body's neurotransmitter channels from brain to muscles are also your pain pathways. We'll discuss exercise or work-induced pain and *non-chronic* pain management in detail later. For now, please accept minor pains as literal Grecian "prices paid" for activity. Sure, this price paid is opposite to the human pleasures we dream about, but *few* of us are totally free of discomfort from arthritis or delayed onset of muscle soreness (DOMS) after our workouts. Or perhaps from mechanical problems of our skeleton or our connective tissues. I think of such uncomfortable feedback as useful signaling to change my actions or behaviors. WebMD offers a quality of life scale for you to (painlessly) consider.[50] You can be a bit **stoic** about pain as a price paid for longevity—yes?

As a stoic, strong specimen, you don't wait, and you don't brag. Consider this:

A strong young construction laborer bragged that he

could outdo anyone when it came to pure strength. He especially made fun of one older worker at the job site. After several repeats of the young guy's rants, the older worker had had enough.

"Why don't you put your money where your mouth is and challenge me to a strength competition?" the elder asked. "I'll bet an entire week's pay that I can haul something in a wheelbarrow over to that building that you won't be able to wheel back."

"You're on, old man. Let's see what you got," the young boaster replied.

The old man reached out and grabbed the wheelbarrow by the handles. Then, nodding to the young man, he said, "All right, hop in."

Do rather than brag. Move metal rather than boast. Mesh your mental thinking and physical doing. Why? You *lift* better when you engage your mind. Honest. Zone **in**, not out when moving stuff. Now Koach, *how much moving is enough?* I'm glad you asked, George. Enough to keep you in the top five to ten percent of your gender and relative age.

Seven main lifts are key to your twice-weekly resistance routines with the *right* weight load to KABOOM.

You can do varieties of all these main moves:

1. Deadlift (for the many reasons cited above)
2. Squat (in many variations)
3. Lunges (also in many variations)
4. Compound thrusters
5. Rows
6. Bench presses or pushups
7. A multi-plane exercise that combines lifting, pulling, and pushing.
   A ten-count bastard routine with dumbbells is one example.

Check YouTube videos or contact your Koach for proper complex moves and protocols.

As you get closer to *stamininety* parties, you logically may drop some routines, and you certainly should adjust loading and ranges of motion to keep on keepin' on. Muscle strength is your natural engine to keep on truckin' whether that strength is applied fast, long or in heavy ways.

Life in Your Fast Lane

When prepared properly, you can complete your intensity-based strength workout rapidamente. You may hear of great "red zone" fast workouts by acronyms of "HIIT" and "SIIT" where high intensity interval and short intensity interval protocols apply. These can be as short (and high) as in four minutes total, thanks to an innovator named Dr. Izumi Tabata.[51]

This periodic technique, which bears his name, is lifting fast in the truest sense! This is heart-thumping, muscle-burning effort. These short and intense strength moves do *not* change one's body composition in a major way. A fast lifting session recruits more of our muscle fibers for intense production and high calorie burn (plus hours of caloric afterburn!). At our ages, we should limit fast lifting routines like Tabatas to *once per week*. Me? I love and don't love 'em as they are *tough*. Precede these short, intense lifting sessions with extra stretching and warm ups. Trust me. *Fast is good for some activities.* Slow hands are good for others.

Mix these three types of strength work. With your trainer (or from self-study), you determine what fast, long, and heavy methods mean for you—at this current time. These parameters will favorably change as you change on your journey. Congrats in advance as you suppress that poverty of flesh and *skinny flabby* condition identified in older distance runners.

Despite any bodily dings or physical conditions, Deb, Garett, George and all of us have *an athlete within* to be the best we can be. Resistance is *not* futile (with my apologies to Star Trek (1996)). Table 1 presents our decent, good and great strength ratings for athletes by decade-age brackets.

Table 1: Strength Ratings by Age

Current Fitness Status or Goal		Boomer General *Decent Deb*	KABOOMER Incremental *Good Garrett*	Competitive *Great George*
Age Bracket	50-60 years of age	1. Ably perform activities of daily life. 2a. Deadlift three quarter of your body weight (one repetition). 2b. Measured Grip Strength is normal for your age and gender. 3. Complete a mile walk/run in 11:00 minutes or less.	1. Ably perform heavier activities before fatigue. 2a. Deadlift more than one times your body weight (1RM). 2b. Measured Grip Strength is strong for your age and gender. 3. Complete a mile walk/run in 8:30 minutes or less.	1. Compete in your chosen activities and finish in top 15 percent for your age group. 2a. Deadlift more than one and one quarter of your body weight. (1RM). 2b. Measured Grip Strength is very strong for your age and gender. 3. Complete a mile walk/run in 7:45 minutes or less.

Current Fitness Status or Goal		Boomer General *Decent Deb*	KABOOMER Incremental *Good Garrett*	Competitive *Great George*
	61-70 years	1. Ably perform normal activities of daily life. 2a. Deadlift two-thirds of your body weight (one repetition). 2b. Grip Strength is normal for your age and gender. 3. Complete a mile walk/run in 9:00 minutes or less.	1. Ably perform all normal to heavy activities of daily life until fatigue. 2a. Deadlift up to one time your body weight (1RM). 2b. Grip Strength is strong for your age and gender. 3. Complete a mile walk/run in 9:30 minutes or less.	3. Complete a mile walk/run in 8:30 minutes or less. 2a. Deadlift up to/more than one time your body weight. (1RM). 2b. Grip Strength is very strong for your age and gender. 3. Complete a mile walk/run in 8:30 minutes or less.

Current Fitness Status or Goal		Boomer General *Decent Deb*	KABOOMER Incremental *Good Garrett*	Competitive *Great George*
	71-80 and "+"	1. Perform most activities of daily life on most days. 2a. Deadlift half of your body weight (one repetition). 2b. Grip Strength is normal for your age and gender. 3. Complete a swift mile walk in 13:00 minutes or less.	1. Ably perform heavy and sustained activities before fatigue. 2a. Deadlift more than your body weight (1RM). 2b. Measured Grip Strength is normal for your age and gender. 3. Complete a mile walk/run in 10:30 minutes or less.	1. Compete in your chosen activity/activities and finish in top 25 percent for your age group. 2a. Deadlift more than your body weight (1RM). 2b. Your Grip Strength is HIGH for your age and gender. 3. Complete a mile walk/run in 9:15 minutes or less.

Table 1 Notes:

1. Biking or swimming may also be used to gauge endured strength levels of distance per time.

   A bridge exists between these endured strength and stamina guidelines. Withered people *don't* walk as quickly as strong folks. (Quicker walkers tend to live longer and better. Yup, slower walkers tend to die younger). Now, what about "us" with physical and/or health challenges? Are we close to dead on arrival? NO!

2. DOA

   Your resistance efforts and strength activities proactively avert or defer your being "**DOA**". **DOA** is our shorthand for **D**iabetic, **O**bese, and/or **A**rthritic conditions that cost many of our peers dearly. Don't be one of "them." It isn't good to be DOA. Yet, it is very good to move objects in *modified* fashion, under the supervision of a professional, when you have a physical (or mental) challenge.

3. Decade Classes

   Right. Decade-aged brackets in our Table 1 are subjective. Many of "us" look to our decade birthdays to take a haj, complete a distance event, or lift a heavier weight for a "personal record." In my experience, achieving a goal or goals simply feels great, and not just as our decade age milestones approach. You do the work, then you celebrate... whenever and wherever you are. Have real fun at seventy-one as well as at seventy!

4. That column category in Table 1 that you classified "as is" today isn't as important as the column that you strive "to be" for your future parties past 90. You are the judge of what and how you lift, push, and pull stuff. Be a great judge, no matter where your court is to preside over heavy objects. And remember endured effort.

Here is one *Don't*, and then one *Do*, for all the Debs, Garretts, and Georges in our generation:

- *Don't* be a victim of that venerable saying: "too soon old, too late smart." Get wise early and get old late, with SAFE strength regimens for moving stuff.
- Do find your vigor. Develop strong shoulders, if able. Brandish weights, as possible. Be the last one dancing past 90. Do take your good strength medicine.

Let's wrap up strength matters and then turn the page to **Stability** as your accident insurance.

One More Time: Be Strang because Strength Matters

A dozen research-based reasons are why a KABOOMER does resistance exercises twice each week. Move stuff about two total hours a week to thrive and strive:

1. Rebuild muscle
2. Recharge metabolism
3. Reduce fat
4. Reduce resting blood pressure
5. Improve blood lipid profiles
6. Resist diabetes
7. Increase bone density
8. Decrease physical discomfort
9. Enhance mental health
10. Revitalize muscle cells
11. Reverse physical frailty
12. Combat cancer.

KABOOM!

BE STRANG—STRENGTH MATTERS— ADDENDA

Four scintillating Strength Addenda follow your ultimate Kool Down chapter.

1. First, you'll ascribe to key safety concerns with "The price is right."

2. You'll reinforce why Strength training is as imperative as medicine.

3. Next, you'll learn more about When? Where? and How? to do your habitual resistance training.

4. And then, as closure for Strength Matters, you'll deliberate on three darned good details:

   • Source Code for Strength

- Muscle Science
- Testosterone and ADAM.

Granted, these Addenda add length to this long read. Yet the direct link of functional strength to longevity and livelihood is vital. Moving stuff serves you well as *medicine*. Exercise over Drugs!

Wither *not* on your uber-important strength journey to party past 90 years young.

CHAPTER 4

KABOOMER
Accident Insurance

I've seen a fall or two, so I can share a thing or two.

Our trusty National Council on Aging offers three sober statistics:

1. A senior is treated in the emergency room for a fall every eleven seconds.
2. Every nineteen minutes, one senior will die from his or her fall.
3. One in four Americans over the age of 65 falls each year.

> *"Falls are the greatest threat to Senior health and safety."*
> —Aging.com

And I quote: "General weakness can...put seniors in danger of seriously injuring themselves in any fall."

This chapter shares critical ways in which you and I can avert injury from falls. Danger Will Robinson! Physical frailty is a danger. You know someone who has fallen; and you know too many who might be seriously injured if they fell. And one-fourth of us Medicare-aged folks *will* fall each year. Take that actuarial statistic to your claim adjuster! Hope is not a stability strategy; rather an *actionable* stability strategy to avert your "greatest threat" is.

Your Insurance Premium

This vitally important section stresses our ability and capability to *avoid* falls by regaining the balance we had as cherubs. Honestly, kids and grandkids can shore up our stability and balance, if we watch 'em and emulate their moves. Have you read that simple things can be hard? Yes, indeed. And should a KABOOMER trip, his or her *retrained* responsiveness can save a trip to the orthopedic surgeon or emergency room. Reflexively and responsively move like a kid and you'll party at 90, without bionic hips or surgically pinned wrists.

Key chapter takeaways for your insurance against accidental injury are:

- Regular balance and stability efforts are *not* demanding. Almost all of us can pursue improved balance and stability.
- Convenient walls, household articles, and the good ol' floor are your insurance allies at prices that can't be beaten.
  - Balancing on one leg is an important test for your brain health (mind-body linkage).
  - Stabilize your *spine* as a baby does. Rock-like bodies do roll (and party).
  - Be proactive with *tune-ups* if/when you develop activity-specific imbalances.

Have I mentioned that you should seek professional clearance to engage in balance and stability moves? Physical aptitude and readiness for us (over age 60) is also a good insurance rider. Get your "PAR-Q" checklist signed!

Kids' Play Means an Accident-Free Day

Think about what most of us did as kids, such as these two playful activities:

1. Carefully and safely stand on one straight leg with both eyes closed and have someone record your standing time.[52]

   "The ability to balance on one leg is an important test for brain health... Individuals showing poor balance on one leg should receive increased attention, as this may indicate an increased risk for brain disease and cognitive decline." - Yasuharu Tabara, Ph.D., Kyoto University Graduate School of Medicine

2. Get down to, and then up from, the ground by yourself and without using your hands or supports. This up and down stability sequence called the Sit to Rise Test.[54,55,56]

Hmmm. Do these two rekindled skills of yesteryear enable stamininety? *You bet.*

- Your timed steadiness with spatial awareness, officially labeled as "proprioception"[57] is Enabler #1.
- Your combined leg strength, coordination and balance to sit and rise is your oft-envied Enabler #2.

Become a KABOOMER who does *not* fall each year. Avoid accidental trips or falls, and/or lessen their "impact" with proper practice at being kid-like or cat-like in reaction. We can and should maintain that stable focus, and train for body responses to slips and trips. Many of us know from the experiences of our loved ones that hip replacements are:

a. Too common,
b. Too expensive, and
c. Avoidable with luck, skill, and your proprioceptive timing.

Ditto for orthopedic pins and plaster casts for fractured wrists. Remember an aphorism about an ounce of prevention in Poor Richard's Almanack? I compliment and complement Mr. Franklin with this stable corollary: an ounce of *proprioception* **prevents** many falls! Say what?

Proprioception

Proprioception is a fancy phrase for our awareness and re-sponsiveness to stimuli. We need to respond to spatial posi-tion, motion, and equilibrium unless we are plants and until we go six feet under. A Doctor Sherrington picked this fancy phrase to mean "one's own reception" a century ago.

Example: If a healthy person is blindfolded, he or she knows through proprioception if one arm is above his or her head or hanging by the side of his or her body. Another instance: Can you lead with *either leg* as you put on your underpinnings, pants, or leggings without experiencing a difference in sta-bility or balance? And here is a another: brushing your teeth using either hand without compromising your pearly whites. Phenomenal football player Odell Beckham, Jr., attributed his equal "handedness" habits, like tooth brushing with ei-ther hand, as one small, simple step toward his millennial fitness. And a fourth habit that I endorse: alternate your lead leg as you climb or descend stairs. In other words, become *more bilateral* in your movement! Most kids know *their own reception*, so most KABOOMERs should regain their spatial recognition and response too. I kid you not.

Fact: Experts state that kids do trip or start to stumble as often we do. Yet their spatial awareness and reactions save them from face-plants, dinged elbows, or worse. As another example: if you can bound up an unknown winding stairway without looking down, your proprioception is probably fair to middling. My dad, a Vermonter, used "fair to middling" to describe how his Greatest Generation life was going on any given day. Here's hope that many of you readers will strive for *more than* fair to middling insurance against falls.

Stability is not a *standalone* element in your wellness (par-don the word selection). Take this to your physical bank ac-count: Stability is directly and deeply linked to your stretch-ing, strength, and stamina efforts for stamininety.

By the Kool Down ending of this book, you will have de-voured all 7S inter-related elements, and you will stand **steady** and tall on your journey, independent of footwear....

How Stable Are Your Silver Sneakers?

Please click on www.silversneakers.com/blog/balance-stabil-ity-exercises-seniors.

Kudos to many Medicare health plan promoters who pro-mote "free" boomer visits to health facilities with Silver Sneak-ers. A freebie? Indeed, for many of us. Guess who does not have Silver Sneaker privileges? Right, your scribe doesn't. That is fine for me, yet I certainly encourage *eligible* folks to get their free gym memberships—and use them.

I have taught Silver Sneaker lessons to my age-grouped peers. I always included major elements of balance and stabil-ity moves to help them put years in their lives. Folks, stability and balance (in any colored sneakers) are *muy importante*![58]

What's our big balance picture? I'm glad you asked.

This chapter's summary figure (below) presents stability *and* balance themes for your consideration and your leverage. I hope you buy into an A+ accident insurance policy to be as stable as possible. *Do* strive for stability and balance, unless of course you *like* free falls, face plants, and hard bounces. If you have a physical condition or need an adaptation for bal-ance and stability moves—there is still something to do—that is to get *started*, baby.

Yes, many stability and balance moves can be traced to baby movements—like a Happy Baby pose. And yes; super stability and balance moves have asana names if you are a yoga prac-titioner. Namaste! Want to be warrior god or goddess? Then use your Wirabhadrasana "warrior" grounded-ness. Your mind-body connection is key.

Options? Become aware of yoga, barre methods, Green Mountain Frosty "homemade" hacks for grounded-ness,

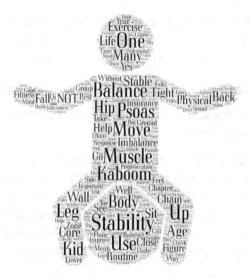

Tai chi or Qi gong. Learn what works for you as you journey toward...you guessed it...stamininety. We won't delve into these tried and true techniques here. You've got a bit of homework if your interest is piqued, and I offer many more thoughts about mind-body alignment in my weblog posts and online presentations. Are you necessarily adaptable?

Adaptation

A quick word about adaptive methods for balance and stability that can be used by folks with Parkinson's Disease (PD). It is very sad, yet very true, that folks with PD "have twice the rate of falls (called PD Falls or PDFs) as their age-matched peers."[59]

This rehabilitation research cites: "The influence of qi gong on postural stability and PRFs was verified.... Qi gong is mindful exercise, a healing component of Chinese medicine, which is congruent with neuroplasticity, brain reorganization, and repair."

Another Adaptation—for MS sufferers

Every Day Health authors advise of the best exercises for those with multiple sclerosis (MS).[60]

An MS sufferer can improve his/her quality of life with balance and stability efforts. See more helpful hints about "Boomers Difficulty with Physical Function" and/or "Needing Help with Daily Activities or Personal Care" at www.prb.org/us-baby-boomers/.

And Another—Scoliosis

Many of us have an irregular spinal shape—or scoliosis. I do. I hope that you appreciate that spinal stability moves help rather than hinder folks with this condition. See what ACE Fitness offers at www.acefitness.org/education-and-resources/professional/expert-articles/5576/exercises-for-scoliosis-how-to-develop-programs-for-clients-with-scoliosis.

Whether we are totally perfect, or whether we have slight or not-so-slight conditions, balance and stability moves are, as the Three Musketeers stated, "all for one and one for all."

Y'all, we must not concede to body stiffness, limited motion, walking aids, safety handrails, and other accoutrements of aging "for other girls and guys." Please note that I *don't* suggest that you or I pursue tightrope walking like a Wallenda.

I *do* suggest that daily stability regimens, as enduring habits, improve your activities of daily life (ADL) and improve your game of chance to avert most falls. I'll argue for your stable fitness with a proverb, scribed by you know who, Richard Saunders:

> "Wise Men learn by others' harms; Fools by their own."—Benjamin Franklin, *Poor Richard's Almanack*

Learn from the accidents, joint replacements and fractures of others! Be a wise and active man or woman; and you will have that priceless accident insurance.

How to begin more stable times?

I mentioned a few new daily habits earlier when I described proprioception. Seven habits to bump up your accident insurance follow.

Step 1. Get a medical professional's up-check.

> Professional "up-checks" are important for gauging possible problems and approving your physical readiness for exercise. *Case*: There is a documented relationship between "poor" balance and the potential for strokes. Yup! American Heart Association "researchers found that those who could *not* balance on one leg for more than 20 seconds had more incidents of cerebral small vessel disease than those who could balance for longer."[61] I do *not* want to spook anyone about strokes. Yet there are very strong correlations between physical aptitude[61] and **lessened** chances for strokes, or diabetes, or "widow-maker" heart conditions.

Step 2. Check your feet, particularly your toes and heels.

> Do you have any limits to "kid-like" ranges of motion? Consciously work these critical footsy elements for your balance and stability.

Step 3. Start with simple, slow heel and toe raises (with both feet on the ground, or with one of your feet on a flat spot of ground).

> Should you have only one operable leg, *please* commit to stable heel and toe raises despite your adaption. Use a safety spotter or stand next to a wall or door surface as a "training wheel" for your lower body lifts.

> Our neighbors to the North (eh) offer many simple and efficient balance moves for seniors.[62]

> Back at home, America's largest lobbying organization, the AARP, also offers many starting routines for balance

and stability. I hope that you'll master these basic balance moves, then progress to more stimulating moves. **Stability matters for making all of your *next years* your best years!**

So Koach, what happens when I reach my candles milestone? My answer is that you **still** move in measured ways to address that Moody Blues' Question of Balance. Check the aging in place website for simple moves to continue as those birthday candles mount: www.aginginplace.org/top-10-elderly-balance-exercises-to-improve-balance-and-coordination/

Step 4. Stand more than you sit each day, every day. Your biggest muscle groups (your quadriceps), and your most powerful muscle group (your glutes or "buns" or "booty") aren't much good if they are kept dormant. You may have heard or read the fitting phrase: "Sitting is your new smoking threat." There is more than a Franklin ounce of prevention in this adage, I assure you.

When you sit; sit tall, as if your belly button is touching your spine. Yes, this is your "deep core" insurance rider *when* it is exercised. Your muscles, connective tissue, and skeleton in your core groups are vitally important to your stability in space! A fancy name for your *core* is *"lumbo pelvic hip complex or LPHC."*[63] LPHC is **more** than your "abs", which some folks call your *core*.

- Please think *deep core*, rather than "just" abdominals when the term *core* is used in this book, or elsewhere. Muscle shape and size do not have to be *seen* to be critical. Yes— "corseted" muscles have strange names—but they *deeply* matter for **spinal stability** and hip alignment/flexion. Press your belly button to your backbone and hold that contraction. A natural corset from your *Internal obliques (IO), Transverse abdominus (TVA), and Psoas* fibers. These groups also counter "dunlaps disease" as in; My belly dun laps over my belt line.

To stay tall & improve your waist to hip ratio – exercise your corset-like deep core muscles!

Step 5. If you do have to sit, get up in a core-centric way. Operationally, this means *get up* as often as possible, *or every 15 minutes* as a prudent rule of thumb. Rise using as little external support or training wheels as prudent for you at that place and time. Use those powerful large lower body muscle groups to rise. A personal training client of mine, a medical professional, says his sure-bet stability check is to see how an adult raises himself or herself from a sitting position.

Step 6. Selectively and safely load your skeleton as a stable platform. *(You will advance to loading your skeleton in unstable spatial moves—but first things first.)*

Step 7. Imagine how you stabilized movements as a kid, then play back to the future. Be kid-like. Enjoy the floor or ground contact, barefoot or not.

Tippy Toes

Repeat after me, please: "Our great [big] toes are *muy, muy importante* for stability and for our ability to move safely."

A recurrent rubric for your stability, in almost every case, is to do smart things daily *to improve your stability and spatial awareness.* Treat your toes, and particularly your big toes well!

Some boomers' great toes are immobile or missing. I know that mine was of limited mobility after I fractured it with an errant kettle bell. My point is this: almost every one of us can engage in full *or* adapted moves to improve our stability.

Can you rise from a chair or not? Extreme physical conditions may impede a small fraction of us from *some* stability routines. Those of us with physical and medical limitations can, with help, benefit from vital, and mindful moves to add years in your life and life to your years. Again, please check with a medical professional to get your official "green light" to engage in balance and stability moves.

Recover, Repeat PRN

Don't just do it; with an apology to Nike's Phil Knight, *Do It Continually!* Do your stability and balance efforts six days a week, twice daily and "PRN" (which is shorthand for a Latin phrase meaning "take as needed"), every week until a doctor says, "Halt!"

Floors, Doors, and Walls

Our baseline, or Zone 1, routines are bilateral; meaning that you use both halves of your boomer body as you balance "on firm ground" rather than on spongy yoga squares, for example. Many of us are "handed" with slight or not-so-slight differences in stability/balance on one side or the other. Intuitively, and as I stated earlier in this chapter, you and I want to be as balanced and stable as possible on "both body sides."

Why? Over-reliance on *bilateral* balancing can mask the subordinate side's capability in relation to the more dominant side.

Improves your balance in "closed kinetic chain" contact with the floor to reinforce "rigidity." That "closed" kinetic chain is considered to be "grounded-ness" by your Koach.

Let's examine a great stability routine, the Wall Sit or Captain's Chair:

Your controlled breathing is a mindful complement to all balance routines. Note to self: Breathe, baby, breathe. In a few days or weeks, you *will* note longer, more stable times. And, you can listen to musical notes of several albums titled "Up Against the Wall" as you build up your accident insurance. In his version, J. Rand sings about working the middle and showing what you got. *Fitting for sitting, Captain?*

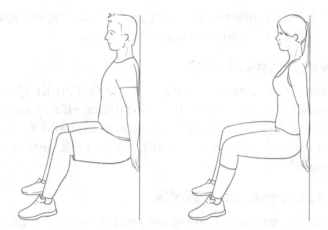

- Be sure to check whether the floor is slippery or slick.
- Stand close to a chosen vertical surface (with your face away). Walk your feet out slowly and safely away from the wall. Just sit for as long as you can. Your quadriceps may be your first stability muscles to hint "uncle."

As your static and core strength permit you, lower your thighs, keeping your shins vertical. If possible, your thighs should be horizontal to the ground.

Think of pushing against the wall, without causing pain to your spinal column. If your clothing "rides up" or if your wall contacts merit a cushion; you can use a yoga mat or foam roller just between "you and the wall".

Enjoy your wall sit until you reach a fatigue point. Celebrate gradual, rigid, and balanced strengthening of your body to hold a position. Go gradually in these steps and progressions, please. This journey isn't a short one, and nor should it be.

Please skip this routine if you are spinal-injured; or modify it as appropriate if you use leg prosthetics. As the resourceful and helpful folks at barbend.com remind us, your quadriceps muscle group is "an important muscle group for *any* success."

This chapter doesn't walk you through *all* the procedural steps for *all* balance and strength exercises that your Koach recommends. Nor does it list *all* the moves in the universe for your grounded proprioception. For your consideration, I offer two options for you to learn and safely execute your progressive moves for balance and stability:

1. If you are inclined to "go it alone," peruse ample YouTube videos and web sources for technique.
2. Consider a personal trainer. He or she can establish bespoke balance and stability routines for you, and then offer prudent progressions.

Progress from basic *rigidity* efforts to more challenging *responsiveness* efforts to the best of your ability. Any and all balance/stability moves enhance your mind-body awareness and your actions in daily life. Right, Grandma?

It *is* a question of balance answered.

Please invest in what it takes for *you* to balance and progressively stabilize your physical 401(k). Yes, you can!

Balanced Trade Tools

Often you may "get what you pay for." Yet, when you consider balance and stability payments and ROIs, that isn't necessarily true. Walls and floors are economical. Prices of these balance and stability items (below) and other apparatus (tools) vary greatly. You might find 'em in your Silver Sneaker "big box" gym if that "price is right," as the legendary Don Pardo offered on radio and television. You might see your trainer unload some of these contraptions from his or her car if you choose in-home training. *You should see what my Toyota Prius can hold when I stage tailored gear for my clients!*

1. Have a *Ball*
   a. with a Swedish "stability" ball (go slow and have a spotter for your safety). Don't let the ball scoot out from under ya in any exercise routine on a stability ball.

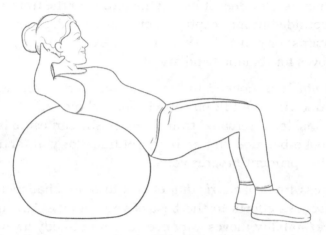

b. Get up on a Both Sides Up (BOSU™) ball or on a Totter Board and be child-like (safely).

2. Try bilateral or single leg rigidity and responsiveness moves on spongy mats/surfaces or yoga cubes.

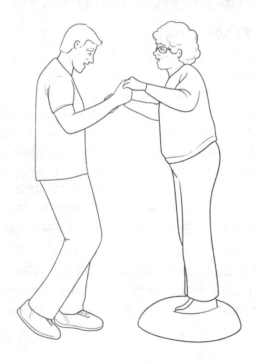

3. Use "functional" exercise slings (e.g., TRX™) and similar suspension straps. Name brand slings can be bit pricey so *caveat emptor* if you are outfitting your home gym. "Generic" stability gear may be just fine.

4. Use a foam roller to support unstable and unilateral balance moves.

5. Floors, Doors and Walls (as already stated and shown elsewhere). These come with your rent or home ownership, right?

I don't have a dog in any fight or chase for fitness equipment sales. You need *very little* new purchases from Amazon or Dick's Sporting Goods or Craigslist to be stable and insured for many moons to come.

"Closed Chains"

This chapter focuses on "closed chain" poses/moves/routines. You guessed correctly —a "kinetic chain" is a linked series of body parts—such as one's hip, knee, ankle, and foot used in a balanced floor move.

Static muscles used to support our LPHC plus knee joints in a wall sit or Captain's Chair (shown earlier) are also a closed chain. As I get older, I find that the value of these closed chain moves is *priceless*. Total resistance exercises suspension straps (TRX straps) are often recommended and used for closed chain movements for strength and stability. Thanks to former Navy SEAL Randy Hetrick for developing TRX for our use! For everything else in fitness equipment and accessories, there *is* a credit card. For relief and function—there are floor, door, and wall *closed chain* routines to do *slowly*.

"Don't worry about upgrading your equipment. **Upgrade** your body."—Anonymous

Sport or Activity-Specific Imbalances/ Instabilities?

Habitual KABOOMERs will likely experience imbalances and/or instabilities on their journey to stamininety. These "come with the territory." I'll drill down into one sport-specific effect from cause as an illustration.

Rowing issues? I assure you from experience, yes, indeed.

Common bodily imbalances and instabilities that come with my "territory" are:

- Quadriceps dominance
- Gluteus muscle weakness
- Hip flexor tightness
- Thoracic kyphosis (rounded upper back)

Sweep rowers (who use more transverse twists to a dominant side) get to enjoy all those, plus one's:

- Outside leg may become stronger than inside leg
- Hips and/or torso become posturally rotated
- Outside arm is stronger than inside arm
- Outside shoulder is posturally elevated compared to inside shoulder.[65]

This list is not intended, in any way, to discourage you from indoor or on-water rowing. *This crew zealot wouldn't do that!* Rather, it *is* intended to remind you that maintenance of your physical 401(k) account includes regular alignment and stability tune-ups. Trust me. One related experience that I will share as your Koach: If you can afford an occasional body massage session, then **go for it**. Proper massages as tune-ups help to mitigate imbalances (and soreness/stiffness), which you may get from life or love or sport. Consider it another investment in your accident insurance.

Can Cycling, Running, or Hiking Also Lead to Imbalances?

You betcha. Most, or all, activities can produce imbalances.

Our posterior chains *tighten*/shorten with pedaling, striding, and walking. If you move your feet, you may have "tight" hamstrings and IT bands, glutes, calves, and/or lower to mid back. Your trainer, physical therapist, or you as a lone ranger/rangerette should *counter* activity-specific problems. I suspect that many of us fall into this usage category. A simple way to lessen posterior chain tightness is simply pedaling in reverse for a short period after a ride.

Fear Not! These tight posterior chain symptoms and triggers *can* be alleviated, but not without not-so-tender, yet loving, attention. Think "strengthen to lengthen" (as you'll read in our Stretching chapter). And think about the Moody Blues in balance.

Proper stability and alignment is important whether you are: 1. "decent" like many of our peers; 2. "better" than most peers; or 3. "best" in your age bracket for performance. Stay aligned and stable; whether you are a walker, rower, cyclist, pickleball participant, or weightlifter.

Drumroll, Please:

1. "The most effective way to address imbalances is through increasing exercise variety and including some additional assistance work;" and
2. "Severe imbalances should always be referred to a medical professional. A qualified physical therapist will be able to identify and correct muscular and postural imbalances."[66]

Note to our stable selves:

"Above all, human existence requires stability, the permanence of things. The result is an ambivalence with respect to all great and violent expenditure of strength."—George Bataille, *Van Gogh as Prometheus*

Human existence needs stability. Yes sir. Yes ma'am. One "deep core" muscle set, which is responsible for flexing our hips in countless moves every day merits your *absolute* attention. When tuned and balanced, the "deep core" psoas[67] matters a whole lot for your permanence. Honest.

Psoas ("SO-az"), Thou Art Our Deepest Stability Secret!

There is only *one* (yup, *1*) muscle group that bilaterally connects our amazing upper and lower body segments. Muscles specifically linking our vertebrae and trunk to our femurs. If you play along with me, look **psoas** up in your dictionary, or please do check what the good Dr. Google prescribes. **Psoas** means "*of the loins*" in Latin.

So, what's the big deal about loins? I can think of several deals. Yet I don't mean what butcher cut is on sale. And what sleepwear you put over your loins is discussed in another chapter. I mean that our **psoas** set is homo sapiens' center-cut or deep core. Some experts assert that psoas are our MVP muscles. If, and when, our loins are aligned, balanced, and supple, life is good. Our upper and lower halves get through daily life without lower back pain, and our spine is stable. When our deep psoas muscle groups are out of whack, our wellness news can take a turn for the worse. Been there, done that.

I once pooh-pooh'ed the lower back issues of others until I had whopper issues of my own! In my defense, I didn't know what *deep core* meant, nor did we know about stretching and stabilizing our loins adequately. Prime professional sport franchises now cater to their MVPs, as well they should. I now pound my bully pulpit for you to work your psoas (also known as hip flexors).

Take care of your MVP muscles, and those loins will take care of you.

I was out of commission for too long when my loins didn't take care of me. Too soon older, too late smarter, I suppose. Get to know your loins (psoas) well.[68]

Want to confirm or deny that you have tight (imbalanced) psoas muscles?

Seven Boomer checks for possible psoas problems:

1. **Leg length discrepancy.**
2. **Knee and low back pain. If you experience knee or low back pain** *with no apparent cause,* it may be coming from your psoas muscles. When your femur is "locked" into your hip socket due to a tight psoas muscle, rotation in the joint can't occur. This can cause your knee and low back torque.
3. **Postural problems**. When your *psoas is too short or tight,* it can pull your pelvis into an anterior tilt, compressing the spine and pulling your back into a "duck butt." If your *psoas is overstretched or weak*, it can flatten the natural curve of your lumbar spine creating a "flat butt." This can lead to low-back injury. You may also feel pain at the front of your hip. Finally, it is possible for your psoas muscles to be *both tight and overstretched.* In this case, your pelvis is pulled forward in front of your center of gravity, causing your back to curve (swayback) and your head to poke forward.
4. **Difficulty moving your bowels**. A tight psoas muscle can be constipating. Yup! Many lumbar nerves and blood vessels pass through and around the psoas muscles. Tightness in the psoas muscles can impede blood flow and nerve impulses to the pelvic organs and legs, and when the psoas is tight, your torso shortens, decreasing the space for your internal organs. This affects food absorption and elimination. As such, it can contribute to constipation, as well as *sexual dysfunction.*

5. **Menstrual Cramps**. An imbalance in a (pre-menopausal) woman's psoas muscles can be partially responsible for menstrual cramps as it puts added pressure on her reproductive organs.

6. **Chest breathing**. A tight psoas muscle can create a thrusting forward of the ribcage. This causes shallow chest breathing, which limits the amount of oxygen taken in and encourages over-usage of your neck muscles.

7. **Feeling exhausted**. Your psoas muscles create a muscular shelf that your kidneys and adrenals rest on. As you breathe properly, your diaphragm moves and your psoas muscles gently massage these organs, stimulating blood circulation. But, when the psoas muscles become imbalanced, so do your kidneys and adrenal glands, causing physical and emotional exhaustion. In fact, according to Liz Koch, author of The Psoas Book, "The psoas is so intimately involved in such basic physical and emotional reactions, that a chronically tightened psoas continually signals to your body that you're in danger, eventually exhausting the adrenal glands and depleting the immune system.[69]"

Are Your Hip Flexors exhausted?

Try this Thomas Test (below) to assess your intimately involved hip flexors.

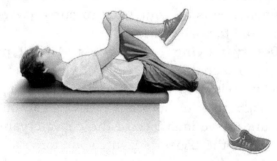

Credit: www.berkeleywellness.com/fitness/injury-prevention/article/get-know-your-psoas-muscles

Koch emphasizes that "our fast-paced modern **lifestyle**— including car seats, constrictive clothing, shoes that throw our posture out of alignment, and more—chronically triggers the psoas." You can visit Ms. Koch's informational website[69] if your KABOOMER interest is piqued.

Yes, stable means "firm" or "steadfast" in our seven-ingredient recipe for KABOOMER fitness and wellness.

Naturally, a stable mind helps with our mind-body cooperation and synergy. Other synergies are highlighted in our Mimic Morpheus (Sleep) and Stress-Not sections to come.

Ready to "upgrade your body"?

Set to be better grounded? Or to show what you got against the wall?

Go. Like the kids we once were. Get firm, then have fun with eyes open or closed.

Keep your Accident Insurance up to date.

CHAPTER 5

The Simple Secret to Lessen Pain and Enhance Gain

"In a wide variety of human activity, achievement is not possible without discomfort."—Malcolm Gladwell, in the foreword for Alex Hutchinson's book *Endure*

Did I quote discomfort? Why, yes I did. Do I underscore KABOOMER achievement? Absolutely. **Stretching** is an *undervalued* and *underused* element of most physical portfolios – perhaps because you have only a tiny bit of discomfort as you allocate your assets. *Value and use* regular stretching. Be flexible to *make your earnings last.* **Even** if your remedial actions bring you close to your "door of discomfort." Your physical 401(k) account is *supercharged* with flexible contributions to lessen pains and grow gains.

You've read about your physical bank's bedrock, **s**tamina. You then read about its foundational cornerstone, **s**trength.

You also absorbed your Koach's counsel about stability as your accident insurance policy.

You will soon read about your daily currency exchange—clean, anti-inflammatory sustenance —to keep your physical 401(k) solvent.

You will soon know why restful sleep—your physical bank's capstone element—is crucial to you.

And you will soon acknowledge what stress thieves can pilfer (or sadly add fat) to compromise your healthy investments. Now, why not indulge in an under-appreciated element of your KABOOMER health?

Stretching complements those other six best practices for your physical journey to stamininety.

Think of our KABOOMER stretches as flexible rate investments in our *lubed, tuned,* and *balanced* physical 401(k) account. As you vary your muscle length and lubricate your joints, you can better withstand variable conditions that you face in life. You make conscious and unconscious decisions about your variable rates of return in your fiscal retirement account, right?

As you extend your partying years, stretching should become a larger asset in our physical portfolio to cope with vital movements (and enjoy life to the fullest). I'm not suggesting that you should become a day trader of variable investments, yet I do advocate your "hedging" against deflation for your physical bank.

Grace DeSimone, a spokesperson for ACSM (the American Council of Sports Medicine) offered: "Your aging body starts calling out for more balanced workouts. Strength and flexibility become major factors.... You've got to oil up the Tin Man." Grab that oil can.

What's the big deal and why the emphases on variable returns in my physical 401(k)? Just spell out S-O-R-E.

Some **O**uches **R**esult from **E**xercise **(SORE).**

If your goal is to *soar* above your peers for fitness and wellness, *soreness* is your shipmate. I reckon that the day I'm not a tad sore is the day that I'm at either Heaven's steps with Saint Peter or at Hell's gate with El Diablo. There is some merit to my high school coach's assertion that "what doesn't smite ya makes ya better."

Shorten Your Injury Recovery

At some point on your journey, you will likely "earn" a physical issue that stretching and flexibility can offset or improve. So, plan ahead. Minimize or mollify this "earned" physical speed bump or detour from perfect travel. A pulled muscle, bursitis, broken toe(s), achy joints, plantar fasciitis…. If you are like your Koach, you've been there, done that. Or you will.

"As you age, you're not only fighting the normal barriers we all have—convenience, transportation, time, environment, weather, lack of enjoyment—but you're also adapting to change," says Stephen Samendinger, Ph.D. "Your body might feel a bit achier than it used to, or your energy levels might take a hit more often than you'd like. These things are completely normal and *shouldn't* stop you from being active—but they often still do."[70]

We will not let minor aches and oomph levels keep us from stamininety, will we? Repeat after me: *We will devote (just right) time to stretching and flexibility regimens to oil-up and to last longer.* Or stated in exterminator terms, we stretch and flex to catch more *mice.*

A Better Mousetrap!

Andy Petranek (a Zen-trained wellness writer) wants you to think about your muscles, joints, and effectiveness as *better mousetraps.* Your "joint is the hinge. For it to work correctly, it needs the ability to fully open, and it needs the spring attached to it to snap it shut…. If the spring you use is too tight, it won't allow the trap to be fully opened, …rendering it (the mousetrap) useless."[71]

I suspect that most of you readers have your own bodily "springs" that are too tight. I do. Rower's elbow is my tight hinge. And it was inferior and hurting!

Loss of precious sleep due to my tingling fingers on my injured arm, four months of bilateral training, a loss of 30 pounds of grip pressure for my injured side, and several *less* inches of arm and shoulder "reach" in a physical therapist's (PT) assessment. I found that out, when I used this Scratch Test coined by a person named Apley.

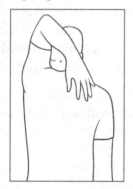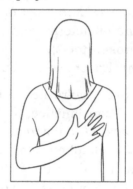

I hope that you will stretch to scratch each scapula, too! Dr. Apley and I will be proud of you.

When a KABOOMER Stretches:

You will *overcome* limitations on flexibility and range of motion by changing:

- Length of muscle fibers, a.k.a. sarcomeres (leading to higher strength as muscle "volume" grows).
- Length of Fascia and connective tissues around stretched muscles.
- Scarred tissues.
- "Gel-like" lubrication of connective tissues—greasing the motion, so to speak.

These benefits are "crucial for maintaining or improving the range of motion of a joint, and in turn minimizing the risk of injury while helping to maximize performance."[72]

- Do you want to feel better as you age? STRETCH.
- Do you want to improve your performance? Flex, and STRETCH properly.

- Do you want to reduce your risk of injury or worse? STRETCH often.
- Do you want to reduce muscle and joint soreness? STRETCH after exertion.
- Do you want to increase your tissues' blood supply and nutrients? STRETCH again and again.
- Do you want a shot at pain-free movements? STRETCH.

Key takeaways for your Stretching and Flexibility chapter are:

- Nearly all of us, despite deficiencies (CP, MS, RA), benefit from regular stretch and flexibility efforts.

- Activities of daily life are better with better mousetraps.

- Habitual stretching and flexibility moves are simple, affordable, and quick!

- Regular and effective stretching and flexibility efforts complement other valuable assets in your physical bank—stamina, strength, stability and even sleep.

- The value of this variable, elastic asset of yours must not be *under*appreciated!

- Know the times when you should *not* stretch.

With these imperatives floating in your mind, let's confirm what stretching and flexibility mean for your physical ROI.

Start at the Beginning

Stretching and flexibility are *not* synonymous with the warm-up and cool-down parts of your regimen. Related? Yes. Synonymous? No. Begin by considering *When? Why?* and *WIFM?* as preludes to your *How* checklists to be like a gumby.

When?

The answer to "When?" is *every day*. Episodic stretch routines after waking up and before bedding down are prudent as we age—daily!

Dan Pink asserted in his book WHEN that one should stretch *when(ever)* you feel like a pliable timeout will help your day.

That could be when you need to warm your muscles to make them more *elastic*, or to prevent injury, or to keep to your routine and enjoy being malleable like our little green friend Gumby from the 1950s. Dan Pink quoted my shirtsleeve relative, poet Robert Frost, who observed: "...the afternoon knows what the morning never suspected."

KABOOMERs are in the daily "know." Know how, and why to bend and stretch.

Why?

Because, sitting is the new smoking. Move. If your activities of daily life involve *any* prolonged periods of sitting—you need to get up, stretch in all 3 body planes, and shake a leg, about every 15 minutes.

Timing may not be everything. Yet timing is certainly something special if you hope to be thriving and striving past ninety.

Muscles and joints have evolved for endured movement—not for desk jockeying. Nor contortions, like this guy:

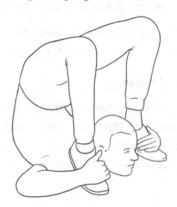

Wow, this is one oiled Tin Man!

However, let's examine effective stretching regimens:

1. **Improve my activity levels!** Plus, I can burn a few more calories, from regular stretching regimens.[61]

2. **Improve my posture!** This is no joking matter, but Artie Johnson quipped: "If God had wanted me to touch my toes, he would have put them on my knees." Not so, Artie!

3. **Manage any back pain and/or arthritis I experience.** One-third(!) of all boomers have osteoarthritis, that "wear and tear" variety of arthritis! "Some people are concerned that physical activity will make their arthritis worse, but joint-friendly physical activity can actually *improve* arthritis pain, function, and quality of life."

4. **Timing!** Author Yuriel Kaim (yurielkaim.com) advises: **"It's never too late** to get your stretch on…. If you're a senior looking to gain more independence, mobility, and flexibility, stretching just might be your new best friend…. Studies have shown that with age, flexibility *decreases by* up to *50 percent* in some joints."[74] We won't let this happen, will we?

5. **If I'm unlucky with MS or CP,** balance-based flexibility moves will help me daily! I may avert prescriptions, assistive medical equipment, or in-home assistants.

Remember – motion is tantamount to life. We're not plants—so we move to live. And limber supple bodies live better!

We're just about to venture into some stretches and flexibility exercises, but keep in mind there are times when you should *not* stretch your body, or a bodily region.

When *not* to stretch a body joint or region

- Your joint lacks stability.
- A bone blocks the motion.
- You recently fractured a bone.
- You have inflammation in or around a joint.

- You have osteoporosis.
- You experience sharp pain with joint movement or muscle elongation.
- You've had a recent sprain or strain.
- You suffer vascular (blood vessel) disorders or skin diseases.
- You suffer a loss of function or decrease in range of joint motion.
- Your joint is hypermobile (large range of motion in the joint).

WARNINGS:

1. If you have any of these "*no* stretch" conditions, do see a sports physiotherapist or sports physician for professional advice before passing "GO." This probably means that you'll miss your $200 Monopoly money on this move, yet it will assuredly pay off in your long game.

2. All stretches present some risk if you use *incorrect* technique or don't follow guidelines or precautions.

   a. Also, some stretches probably should not be used by average or novice athletes – until they are ready. The World's Greatest Stretch (WGS)[75] is one such stretch.

   b. As a counter-intuitive, some common exercises can be detrimental to conditioning programs for specific sports (I know this from rowing).

Play Doctor for Flexibility

Ask yourself:

- What does this joint normally do?
- What is its range of motion, both active (client moves it) and passive (your trainer moves it safely)?
- How is my unaffected side in comparison (if applicable)?

See meded.ucsd.edu/clinicalmed/joints2.htm for many assessments of joint mobility and utility. Selected *Trouble Spot* **stretches** that I use are:

1. **Neck**

   Our noggins are like a very heavy weight on a rather slender support pole—and unless you're Hulk Hogan, you **should** do neck flexibility moves often. One that works for me at episodic intervals through each day is what I call the *Turtleneck*. Extend your neck forward for about two seconds, then tuck it back for about two seconds— your many muscle groups supporting su *cabeza* will feel better!

   For our boomers who are currently "inflexible" or suffer from a stiff or movement-impaired neck, the Silver Sneaker program offers this to help you:

   > Stand or sit in a sturdy chair with your feet flat on the floor about shoulder-width apart. Turn your head slowly to the right until you feel a gentle stretch. Make sure not to tip your head forward or backward. Hold for 10 to 30 seconds, then turn your head to the left. Repeat three to five times[75].

2. **Shoulder Girdle**

   Stand with your feet shoulder-width apart. Hold one end of a towel in your right hand. Raise and bend your right arm to drape the towel down your back. Keeping your right arm in place, reach behind your lower back and grasp the opposite end of the towel with your left hand. Now, you should be holding the towel with your right hand behind your neck and your left hand behind your lower back. Gently pull the towel down with your left hand. You should feel a gentle stretch; but stop if you feel pain. Do three to five times. Switch hands so your left hand is behind neck and your right hand is behind lower back, and then repeat.

   And, you can contact your Koach for personalized stretching regimens.[76,77]

Frozen?!

With my family name of Frost, I should cite a reference for frozen shoulders also:

www.verywellhealth.com/how-do-i-know-if-i-have-a-frozen-shoulder-2696429

Lumbo Pelvic Hip Complex (LPHC)

As mentioned, a LPHC is four-letter acronym for your CORE. Your "centroid" muscles, connective tissue and skeletal bones are vital for KABOOMER stamininety!

Lower Back!

Sit toward the front of the chair with your feet about shoulder-width apart and flat on the floor. Keeping your neck and back straight, slowly bend forward from your hips. Slightly relax your chin and neck. If you can go a little deeper, continue bending your body toward the floor, and slide your hands down your legs toward your shins. Hold for 10 to 30 seconds, then slowly straighten up until you are in the starting position. Repeat at least three times.[78]

Hips!

Comprehensive hip assessment details can be viewed online: meded.ucsd.edu/clinicalmed/joints5.htm. Gain a *good* range of hip motion, as this linked site mentions!

If you're an *angle* aficionado, "the hip is a ball and socket type joint, formed by the articulation of the head of the femur with the pelvis. Normal range of motion includes abduction 45 degrees, adduction 20-30 degrees, flexion 135 degrees, extension 30 degrees, internal and external rotation. Hip pathology can cause symptoms anywhere around the joint, though frequently pain is anterior and radiates to the groin region." Keep your hips away from pathology, okay?

Now, let's consider the principal joint between our leg bones: the knee. The word origin for "knee" traces to "agile, and kneeling." I need not dwell on how critical (and frustrating) our knees can be. Nor do I need to chat about how many "bionic" and expensive knee replacement surgeries are done on baby boomers. Keep your principal leg joints stable and mobile so that you can kneel, bear crawl and frolic with your grandkids like I do.

Knees!

Assessing "normal" ranges of motion for this complex joint's musculature and connective tissue is best appreciated by viewing this UC San Diego medical site. So many knee problems can be traced to our ancestors as they opted to move on two legs! I advocate strengthening and balancing the frontal quads and posterior hamstrings to alleviate "some" knee issues as a first order of business. After all, these major skeletal muscles support such a key part of our skeleton! The NFPT[79] reminds us that "Knee pain and complaints are common" due to this joint's complex structure and heavy use. Oy—even KABOOMERs are not immune.

How snappy a mousetrap is each of your knees? Get snappy (and oiled), please.

Ankles, Lower Legs, and Feet?

Can anyone spell Achilles pain or plantar fasciitis? Your Koach would rather that you spell **fasciitis** than experience it! Trust me.... Though often associated with runners' stresses,[80] many non-runners can also experience plantar fasciitis issues that last and last, regrettably.

I invested plenty of time and effort on my "wheels" in my earlier days chasing Phidippides. These wheels weren't steel radials, and they needed to roll in all weather conditions. Do not let lower extremity dings or pains become chronic or severe. Be proactive and...play.

Playtime

Todd Hargrove's new book, *Playing with Movement*,[81,82] underscores how "the most capable movers—kids, animals, and athletes—develop skill and movement through **play**." Sounds like that challenge we pondered in our Stability as Accident Insurance Chapter, doesn't it? By making some of the physical movements that kids/grandkids (if not animals) and athletes do, **we can** be the last ones partying at 90.

Ever watch pre-game, or pre-race, rituals of professional athletes? These are not slam-bam quickie events. They are habitual moves to warm up muscles and joints, and to tune one's spatial awareness (proprioception) to upcoming game conditions.

Experts say that your *dynamic* warm-up period may beneficially include "some" of your actual exercises to get lubed and ready for action. Many of my crew colleagues spin on indoor rowers before getting on the water to raise their heart rates and limber up to limit chances of injury. I spent most of my time, before getting "hands on" with a crew shell, on *dynamic* stretch routines. I start with my smaller muscle groups and joints—neck, forearms—then shift to my core and lower body. Different sports or activities have similar warm-up progressions and bespoke additions. Walkers, for instance, may include lower-leg shin stretches if they sense that shin splint conditions are a-callin'. My purpose in dynamic stretching is to get fluid in motions relating to all three of my body planes. Note: longer duration *static* stretches *of 15 or more seconds* should be saved until *after* your workout or activity.

Which Moves? I add lunge-twist moves and reverse wood chops to this nice Health.com[83] series of seven (7) pre-workout stretches you might want to consider. I don't wear tights that look like those pictured on that website—by the way.

I implore you to start and sustain your habitual stretches. *Be ready for your long game of life and play.* And never think that you're a Lone Ranger or a Solo Rangerette. Friends, like Tonto, can support ya.

You've Got a Friend - Therapy

Consider adding maintenance massage sessions—if you can afford them, and if you can find those *magic* massaging hands and fingers that make you melt.

Consider relaxing, warm baths to "let it go" (and improve your restful sleep if you complete your dip 60-90 minutes before your pillow time). What if you need to pull a *Trigger*?

Trigger Point Therapy

Trigger points (which you can feel with your finger touches) are taut, kinked, and irritable muscle fibers that affect one's range of motion. The cause of that irritation point may be *that* muscle group, or a "referred" pain from another muscle or connective tissue—perhaps your neck or back. I have no intent to give "TMI" or to "trigger" a lecture on physiology. However, rolling, massaging and kneading efforts by you or a "helper" should *not* cause you pain or intensify the pain that you have from sore muscles or connective tissue (fascia). Listen to your pain meter and stop short of that *door of discomfort* for muscular, fascial, and referred irritations, okay?

Here's another big word with big implications for stamininety – *myofascial. Myo* is the old root word for muscle and *fascia* is the old and new word for our connective tissue.[84]

"Please release me, let me go," as Engleburt Humperdinck sang. I nominate this still-performing gent from Madras, India, as a honorary *humperdincking* KABOOMER.

True, there is professional debate about the value and merits of myofascial efforts. Do I feel that myofascial release methods work? Yes, they work for me, and my hourly rate for self-massage is low. Many of my clients who exercise "hard" also find that these methods help them to be better mousetraps. As my rule of thumb, if you find a motion that aggravates your sensation from a trigger point, you can also find a movement to ease the irritation. Hence, let it go with myofascial releases that you can do all by your lonesome.

Self -Myofascial Releases (SMR)

Deep Recovery folks offer informative Why? What? and How? videos at deeprecovery.com/videos/. YouTube offers many others to help get folks attuned to what these "self-made" relief motions can and should do for you.

Have a Ball!

I stock small, medium, and large game balls to help me release trigger points: *Golf balls* for foot rolling, *Lacrosse/field hockey balls* for my shoulders and arms, and *Softballs* for larger areas like my IT bands. I advocate longer (36-inch) and firmer "foam" rollers so that your entire spine can be supported. Or "rolling" long troublesome IT bands [on the outsides or distal parts of your upper leg].

The walls and floor around you are your self-release friends. These "stand-by" or "flake-out" surfaces are cheap and effective tools to get your muscles un-triggered. It may take a few days to get your sore points or trigger areas released. Yet when you do, it is almost heaven.

Returns on Investment (ROI)

What are variable assets for *stretching and flexibility* practices?

Your ROI from Habitual Stretches and Flexible Practices

1. Your Mousetrap works far better with improved ranges of motion and joints that bend and twist! And your own good posture inspires others to be like you.

2. **Find harmony in your Mind-Body connection plus indomitable Spirit.** We refresh our mindful connections touch with ourselves and our intents.

   Yoga or other "mindful, relaxing, breath-centric" practices shush our minds' busy signals, improve our functional capacity to live well, and help us mind-meld our spiritual intentions and goals. Quiet poses and pranayamas (which in Sanskrit means breath-controlling efforts) can work wonders for you, as they do for me, even if I don't know proper asana labels. Note: My certifying body for professional training, the NFPT, offers a nice summary of what yoga techniques can do to benefit nearly all of us:

"Yoga...centers the body; with autonomic balance, homeostasis occurs, and practitioners experience enhanced coordination.[85]"

3. **Reduce your Body's and Mind's Stress and Tensions. You can get past your demi-hassles or daily life and, repeat after me**—*relax!* Relaxations help you and me manage our stress, strain, and discomfort or pain. Our primal brains are wired for the four F's: food, fight, flight, and f@#$. Can hard-wired adrenal functions be eliminated? No. So, our flexibility program habits can mitigate that hard-wiring. We can stretch to quell physical and mental stressors in our lives.

4. **Know Yourself in new ways.** Our improved flexibility gives us something to struggle against and lean into—mindfully. Flexibility practice stretches more than our muscles. We expand our minds too, by stretching that *muscle* between our ears!

5. **Improved Posture and Body Symmetry. Yes, I endorse the adage "sitting is your new smoking."** *Can you say, "I quit" or "I'll break up my sittings"?* Your flexibility will help you stand taller and longer, plus sit better with expanded *ergonomic* awareness.

6. **Improve your blissful restorative Sleep.** Your stretching routines, before nappucinos or restful sleep *do* help. I speak from my countless experiences. Your habit-forming stretches and/or breath-centric yoga moves (even if you can't pronounce or spell *pranayama)* reduce stress,

relax the body and mind, and improve overall sleep fitness.[86]

7. **You'll feel better in the morning. One of the greatest benefits of daily flexibility routines is your** *joy* factor. It feels good to do something good for the body and the mind. Stretching can reenergize you and keep you on your journey.

Après Activity—your Static Stretches

Remember to invest in static stretching *after* workouts or activity (like après ski). For once, a term of our trade is self-explanatory! Static.... Again, do *not* skip these stationary and slow stretches after your workouts, please—unless your gym or boathouse has a fire alarm. Here's a Canadian journal's rationale:

> **"You should not try to permanently improve range of motion with extensive stretching in your warm-up, just like you would not try to get stronger by lifting heavy weights in a warm-up."**—David Behm, PhD.

Got that? So—these longer duration and non-motile stretches are designed to improve your range of motion and flexibility—over time (of a few days or weeks). I've read of varying time durations as "optimal" to attain your flexibility goals. Some experts have shared 20 seconds for a "hold." Other sources suggest static holds of about a minute. See what works for you, as every KABOOMER is different, some closer to Gumby than I am. Find your secret stretch recipe for essential stretches, post-exercise. Below, I list key static stretches; and illustrations and procedures can be found at my wellpastforty.com site. Also, you can always call me as your Koach for instructional tips.

Stretch examples

1. *Quadriceps*
   Lying on your right side, pull left heel into left glute, feeling the stretch in the front of the thigh. Repeat with the right leg. You can also stand on one leg and safely pull your other bent leg behind you by holding your ankle.

2. *Hamstrings*
   Lying on your back, lift and straighten one leg directly above hips. Holding the calf or thigh, press heel toward ceiling as you pull leg back toward chest. Then switch legs. You may use a "yoga band" (or another accessory like a jump rope) to help with static stretching.

3. *Glutes*
   Lying on your back, cross right leg over bent left knee. Then bring left knee to chest, holding onto the back of your thigh, gently pressing right knee wide. Switch legs.

4. *Chest*
   Standing straight, interlace fingers behind your back as you straighten out your elevated arms and lift your chin toward the ceiling.

5. *Triceps and shoulders*
   Take one arm overhead, bend at elbow joint, and extend palm down the center of your back, gently pulling your elbow with opposite hand. Then, take that same arm across the chest, gently pulling at the elbow joint to extend through the shoulder. Switch arms.

6. *Core and back*
   On all fours, round out your back (like an angry cat), and then invert it, making a C-shape with your spine. Repeat three times. Then sit back between your heels, with forehead on the mat and arms extended in front of you, as you lengthen your back. A "***child's pose***" is a wonderful stretch. So is the pigeon pose below, with our inscribed stability themes.

Your Flexible Account

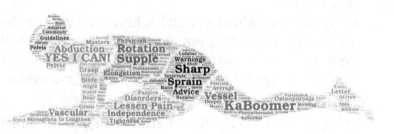

Bottom line – KABOOMERs *invest* in regular stretching. **Period.**

Personal Trainers and kinesiologists use the term *chains* to connect or link muscles groups associated with movement. We call our "backside" grouping of muscles and connective tissue our *posterior chain*. Elements of our posterior chain stretch from our heels to our neckline through our back and spread from hip to hip and shoulder to shoulder. As an example, a dead(weight) lift or deadlift focuses on the muscles and connective tissues (and bones) in our posterior, more than the frontal plane, which I call the toes-to-nose plane of our bods.

Guess what sitting does to most of us? Yup—tight hamstrings. You *must* counteract the contracted condition of posterior muscle groups by stretching. If you move your feet in many healthy strength and endurance moves—you may have "tight" hamstrings and IT bands, glutes, calves, and lower/mid backs. This muscle and fascial tightness is acknowledged as a cost of developing stamininety. I *also* welcome your efforts to get those kinetic rubber bands *loose* and *un-kinked*, as a "variable" investment in your physical 401(k) account!

Fear Not! These tight, posterior chain symptoms and triggers *can* be alleviated, but they need your not-so-tender attention. Tenderloin? "Loin" in Latin is *psoas*. I have trouble with Latin, like Dan Quayle. Luckily, I don't have current trouble with my loins.

You know how important your limber and lubed loins are. You may realize what's at stake to avoid or mitigate lower back pain or something worse. You've already read that, "sitting is the new smoking." So, move often to shift from evil sedentary slouches at desks or in cars: **don't** sit more than necessary. *Prevention aces* aches, pains, and remedial cures! Poor Richard advised us so.

Note: Many sources and folks use the synonym *"hip flexor"* in place of our psoas muscle pairs, and that is fine. After all, hip flexion is what your tuned *psoas* muscles *do*. Or what they *don't* do if these hidden important muscles are stressed or tight. Flex and stretch *your hip flexors (and supporting core muscle groups) each, and every day.* Some sources suggest that our tuned-up psoas muscles relate to major health matters stretching beyond fitness—as Dr. Northrop contends on her website.[87] I bet two nickels that both men and women appreciate the merits of hip-hinging motions.

Pain in the Butt

Please take a little web safari or check with Dr. Google for the amazing maze of muscles and connective tissue in your and my derriere. Amidst those powerful three vertical gluteal muscles is a horizontal muscle fiber that has often given me a pain in one "cheek" or in both. With heavy strength and work, this relatively minor muscle, with another funky Latin name for "pear-shaped"—*piriformis*—can give you out-sized discomfort. In fact, this muscle even has a syndrome named for it—wait for it...piriformis syndrome.

Have you had one of those syndrome experiences like I have? When these muscles are tuned, our femurs move better. Yeah. When they are not tuned, or are stressed or inflamed, their proximity to our $#%^& sciatic nerves can be a painful condition. When I experienced quasi-religious sciatic nerve pains with my very own pains in butt for the first time, I self-diagnosed them as my personal piriformis syndrome. A life-changing orthopedic surgeon set me straight, after fusing my L5-S1 disc herniation. But you scanned that story in our KABOOMER introduction. Thank you, Dr. Moitoza!

Are there good and proper stretches and activities to lengthen, strengthen and ease stress on these piriformis muscles? Yup. Get to know them, (via self-study or by tapping a personal trainer or physical therapist) and use them before a pain in butt strikes you. Okay?

After nattering at you about the whys, dos, and don'ts of flexibility and stretching, you might appreciate some "hacks" that have helped my peers and me perform better.

I say again... *stretching is wonderful for avoiding injury;* stretching is affordable; and you can and should stretch throughout your days – from commutes, to work or play, to exercise, to pre-pillow times. Got it? Are strength and stretching efforts related to stamininety? You bet, Red Rider!

Strengthen to Lengthen

If you're one who likes to take things to the limit; yes, you might be able to *over*-stretch, *over*-roll, or *over*-release your tight *knots.* Yet that is rare, in my experience. If a slight runner invests a lot of effort rolling his or her "IT bands"—the outsides of upper legs from our Ilia (hip) to Tibia (lower leg)—it may be possible to overdo those stretches or rolls. My pushback in this possible scenario goes back to the *"Strengthen to Lengthen"* adage. Thicker, slightly more muscular IT regions are less likely to get aggravated by massaging and/or rolling for *release.*

Rockin' and rollin' accessories for stretching to improve flexibility include:

1. *Firm* cylindrical rollers (either smooth-surface, or nubby)
2. Sized round objects (golf balls, field hockey or lacrosse balls, and baseballs/softballs)

3. Stretch bands (*be careful as they do wear out and they can snap*)
4. Stability ball.

Yes, we experience "*tightness*" caused by muscular micro-tears and inflammation in our connective fascia after exercise. We can use (all by ourselves) simple round objects to release knots and to smooth fascia in order to perform at our best. Big muscle groups need their releases, I assure you. And, DOMS, for **d**elayed **o**nset of (your) **m**uscle **s**oreness can be mitigated. This I hope that you get! And golly again...I wish that I had used stability balls, bands and firm rollers in my days of yore. Too late smarter for release.

Please Release Me, Let Me Go...

Unkink your temporary kinks or scar tissue to KABOOM.

"Foam rolling can be used immediately before exercise to increase flexibility, particularly as there seems to be no adverse effect on athletic performance. Regular use may also improve flexibility long-term. Foam rolling can also be used in the short-term after exercise to reduce the sensation of muscle soreness."[88]

Plus, "Self-myofascial release may reduce perceived soreness and increase pressure pain threshold as a result of DOMS during the 48 hours following damaging exercise."[88]

Here's Teddy Roosevelt's and my bully-pulpit: Get a foam roller and some hard, round things into your arena! Or look like a cat.

Consider, then assume a "good" **cat pose** (www.yogicwayof-life.com/marjari-asana-the-cat-pose/). Just imagine a black cat with its arched back around Halloween time. Or if you know Sanskrit, imagine this routine as a *marjariasana*. I speak from my practical, all-fours-on-the-floor, and slow-it-down experiences, that the c**at** does indeed: 1. help my spinal stability; 2. lessen my back fatigue from its flexing; and 3.

lengthen parts of my MVP *core*. Ha, I did a closed chain yoga pose and I didn't know what an *asana* was.

Functional, closed-chain exercises like the CAT recruit more of our muscle groups and require additional skeletal stabilization with our arms and/or feet on the ground.

You may be more used to *open-chain* moves in a gym, like machine-based leg exercises, or bench presses—and that is fine. Just add *closed-chain* routines to your repertoire. Why? Athletes can better their skills (like throwing a baseball at higher speed) with closed chain moves. Would the good folks at Sparta Science lie to you and me? I think not. See this *Closed Chain Exercise is Critical* web post.[89]

I know what you are pondering, so here's my response before you raise your virtual hand. Yes, indeed; there are useful "open kinetic chain" routines that co-improve our stretches and stability when we want to, or when we need to isolate one muscle group. You see, strength and stability/stretch moves are complementary for both rehabilitation and fitness gains. Check 'em, embrace 'em, and benefit from 'em in your regular, combined protocols. Please contact your trainer or call your Koach for good 'ol "open" moves to help you party past 90.

What is Old Is Again New

Honest Abe offered this thought which is relevant to your stretching and flexibility habits:

> "...as the cause is new, so must we think anew and act anew."

I *think and act in new ways* to improve my variable investments and prospects for stamininety. How about you?

That is a wrap for your *basic* KABOOMER stretching and flexibility. The more flexible you are (to a limit), the better you can enjoy your activities of daily (and nightly) life. And, the more you will be able to be the life of the party at ninety. Don't be too kinky, and don't be stiff (with one possible exception). Stretch and roll daily as your variable investment for stamininety. Act anew to make *stretching* and *flexibility* a key component of your supercharged physical 401(k).

CHAPTER 6

Stress Steals Years and Cheers

"Old age isn't so bad when you consider the alternative."—Actor Maurice Chevalier

Stress is a *life-threatening* and *life-shortening* force in our older ages. That is, unless you act. Unless you layer your defenses to counter that badly behaving chemical force within you. **Stress Steals!** It can pick your life's pocket, steal your health card's PIN, or get access to your physical safe deposit box. Cheer up, KABOOMER. Enjoy an alternative of chill and mellow. Act to counter Stress for years to come.

Paraphrasing Charles Dickens: Let us savor springs of hope, and view winters for what they are. We are blessed to have good years before us.

"Chronic" stress is *conversely* linked to your and my sustenance, stamina, strength, and restorative sleep. Yes, stretching and stability efforts are adversely impacted too. You must whip stress and "whip it good..." (thank you, Devo).

Takeaways for this thievery chapter are:

- You can watch things happen, or you can *make* sunny things happen.

- Laughter is munificent medicine, even if your joke went over like a lead balloon.
- Anti-inflammatory habits in diet and exercise - *do* work to lower cortisol and stress levels.
- Breathing *boxes out di*stress. Think of "breath taking" efforts to counter theft.
- Ninety-five percent of life is small stuff. *Don't* voluntarily sweat small stuff. Do de-tension. Loosen up.

Stress Defined

Medical experts label stress as "a physical, mental, or emotional factor that causes bodily or mental tension. Stresses can be external (from the environment, psychological, or social situations) or internal."

Cunning linguists know that the word origin of stress is the Latin "strictus" which means drawn tightly. Old English and French derivations are also provocative. Old English roots[90] are "distress" and "strict," or a "hardship or force exerted on a person." The French root? "oppression."

Are any of these body parts: brain, muscles and joints, heart, stomach, pancreas, intestines, and reproductive glands important to you? I'll wager that your answer is yes. Our minds and bodies are (strictly) drawn tight and put in distress in response to hardships we experience. Fend off French oppression!

Perhaps you already know that:

- Stress can *adversely* impact your sexuality and performance.
- Your gut is impacted by stress.
- Stress raises your tension and blood pressure.
- The mental weight of our wacky world can make your joints ache.

Oy! There are physical, mental and emotional assets that can be stolen...if you or I let the thief into our physical bank account. I'm keen to avoid time bandit thefts, and I trust that you will too.

Are You Stressed or Chill?

Find out for yourself. Try this Stress Quiz: ndstate.co1.qualtrics.com/jfe/form/SV_78qiyDZgnHZG7OZ

Or consider smartphone or web applications to catch your thief and put him or her away in jail: www.ag.ndsu.edu/nourishyourbody/apps-to-reduce-stress.

Where the F*ck did Stress Come From?

Life happens, or as we said in my naval career, Ship Happens. Leading a team for 133 hours in an abnormal "work week" happened to me. Handling and safeguarding a tiny portion of our nation's nuclear arsenal happened to me as a leader at age 22. Helplessly listening to 9/11/2001 news accounts from London happened to me. Yes, ship happens to all of us! Stress comes from many external sources. Yet, KABOOMERs do not let *distress* grow too much, too fast from *internal* triggers.

Stress is ingrained, and it is intertwined with many activities of your and my daily lives such as: work, play, romance, kids, grandkids, and interactions with rude folks. Few of us would be here today if the *fight or flight* responses of our primordial brains didn't kick in before saber-toothed tigers grabbed us.

If a bully did more than kick sand in your youthful face, you probably reacted to a "put up your dukes" trigger from that primal brain. Ladies? If you ever saw a child of yours step off a curb and into traffic, that most assuredly triggered a stressful response. Our evolved brains are wired to trigger our: 1. fight, or 2. flight, or 3. feed, or 4. *frolic* (a slightly modified fourth "F" for primal thoughts and actions).

How did we Baby Boomers evolve our stress mechanisms? And why does our sympathetic "reptilian" brain do what it does? Just spell after me: S-U-R-V-I-V-A-L.

Imagine for a moment that you are splashing in the California surf. You see a great white shark headed your way. Your reptilian brain elevates your adrenaline to fight-or-flight response quicker than you could scream "shark"! It triggers you into a "F" action, when in extremis.

Sure, my dolphin brain (frontal lobe) wants me to communicate, travel widely, build social skills, and eat well; and those activities are good things. Yet my primal pleasure brain likes other useful "feel good" activities, if you get my train of thought and recall the fourth F. Does this have anything to do with stress? Si.

All Stress Is Not Generated Equally

Recall that we're here today because fearsome felines didn't catch our Paleo predecessors.

Let's quickly clarify the types of *stress* we want to minimize or avoid. That type is *Extended Distress* which can become chronic or permanent. Each of us has experienced performance gains following short-term beneficial stress (butterflies, pre-game jitters, or a bit of adrenaline when needed to get that medal or prize).

Repeat after your Koach: We *need the right type of stress for short performance* periods. Are you an adrenaline addict who wants to run with the Pamplona Bulls, bungee-jump from a tall bridge over troubled water, or swim among Amazonian piranhas? If so, go for it.

Yet it's best not to spend *all* your days pulsing your adrenal and endocrinal glands. That is, unless you want to heighten your prospects for *bad* chronic and acute thieves like high blood pressure, poor moods, high estrogen, loss of muscle mass, and loss of (grey) matter in your brain. It's a *no brainer* to state that *excess* alcohol or drug ingestion (regardless of our cannabis lobby) is unhealthy stress. Honest.

Remember Devo's "whip it good" words. Develop your *stress not* game plan, which help you party past 90. Be proactive rather than reactive!

"Stress doesn't kill you. **It's your reaction to it.**"—Hans Selye

Before I offer antidotes to adverse reactions, let's play a game of Truth or Consequences. Though I won't pressure you...

Truth or Consequences

Our endocrine systems secrete **Cortisol**,[91] "...a steroid hormone, produced by the adrenal cortex, that regulates carbohydrate metabolism, maintains blood pressure, and is released in response to stress."

In my Koaching terms, cortisol adversely impacts both protein synthesis and our normal responses to inflammation and immunity. Cortisol is also related to weight gain. Please don't think that our temporary application of hydrocortisone ointment for bug bites or rashes is all "bad." Rather, truth is our bodily cortisol secretions from chronic (extended) distress can lead to bad effects like these:

- A rise in blood sugar and blood pressure.
- Lessened immune system resistance to infection; and
- *Early cell aging.*

*Chronic stress equals **early aging.*** Chronic stress equals a shorter life and eclipses one's chances to party past 90! And that's the Truth! That early aging is thievery! Do not raise such a thief or suffer unwanted consequences.

Are Life Stresses Raising Your Cortisol?

Why not check on your potential "silent killer"? Your subjective survey findings may enable lifestyle changes that promote stamininety.

1. This first survey is brought to you by The American Institute of Stress: *www.stress.org/self-assessment/*

2. Next, is a *Personal Well-Being Survey:* www.heartmath. org/resources/personal-well-being-survey
   This online Survey has 25 questions and only requires 4-5 minutes to complete. I don't want you to stress-out on this—just take it.

3. And third, your Koach suggests this **Holmes-Rahe Life Stress Inventory.** Your free limited-use template is located at www.familyofmen.com/wp-content/uploads/2012/04/stress_scale.pdf.

What are the big deals and stressors for us? At the top of our list is loss of a loved one or loss of your livelihood.

Oy! Loss of a loved one. Chris Erksine wistfully wrote in one *Los Angeles Times* column after his beloved wife passed.[92] KABOOMERs, like Chris, like you and me, should face everything in their Middle Ages, and rise, when they can, after sad or tragic loss.

FEAR is False Expectations Appearing Real

Better yet, remember that **you** can *"Face Everything and Rise."* That alternative acronym for FEAR is a good mantra to help you and me keep on keeping on and fearing *not.*

Rise like a phoenix. Then, rise higher and higher as you prepare to party past 90, thriving and striving as you go.

Three related ways to face everything in stride are: resilience, perseverance, and grit.

1. *Resilience* is your ability to bounce back after adversity or disappointment; and it is being able to manage and adapt to sources of stress or adversity. (I mentioned the importance of bio-resilience in another segment.)

2. *Perseverance* is your steady mastering of skills or completing a task, while having a commitment to learning.

3. *Grit* is a more recently authored term for Face Everything and Rise, as researched by Angela Duckworth. Grit is defined as the tendency to *sustain* interest and effort toward long-term goals. It is associated with self-control and deferring short-term gratification.[93]

Bounce back. Erksine grittily did. You can too, though no one said this was a walk in the park. We are steadfast in our daily pursuits and lifelong learning. We keep on keepin' on, rising toward our long-haul goal to live longer and live better.

Cope and counter! Yes—you can, with grit, humor, fresh air, friends, exercise, and—the fourth F. Yes—you can—like a celebrity without a major care in your world. You can take proactive security steps to counter stressful vitality thieves.

Moderating or mitigating stress is simply hard, despite our recognition that thievery is bad for us and for those we love. *Why?* We get caught up in life. We don't know how to say No. We think we're pretty good at burning candles at both ends. We forget how to be playful.

A simple thing of importance for your physical 401(k); reducing your stress levels and the occurrences of stress—is - simply stressful.

Do *not* stress. Benefit from these healthy habits:

a. Regular seven hours of restful sleep
b. Warm mineral baths
c. Chuckling 'til we are buckling
d. Mindful breathing.

Distress is an issue of severity for many born between the years of 1946 and 1964. Few Boomers find the time, or invest their "invaluable" time, to be playful. Else, your epitaph may read:

"Here I lay before my proper time.
I guess I worked a lot of overtime.

My goal was, little things, to never blunder,
Unfortunately, that put me six feet under."

Let's get specific with ways to avoid pilferage of your vitality from chronic stress, as suggested in this chapter wordcloud:

Hold Stress at Bay with Play

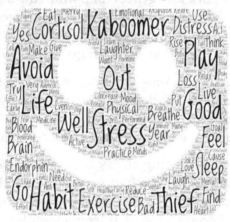

Note that shades of blue are deemed to be our most relaxing colors. **Enjoy blue skies, blue paperback covers, and stress *not*.**

Fear not, and stress not. Your Koach counsels you to *side-step* synthetic versions of what your body can produce naturally. Prescribed meds, such as sedatives, just might cause more problems than they solve! Actively avoid downward spirals that boomer peers you may know are experiencing:

A depressed, stressed elder feels down and/or anxious. He or she takes prescribed pills and feels a bit better for a short time. Regrettably, that boomer senses a need for more and more pills to get the same desired effect. Reliance on meds may cause deeper swings on this downward spiral. No matter the fault(s), the spiraling matter is epidemic to our generation and nation! Polypharmacy.

In contrast, a KABOOMER chooses to exercise. She or he puts in a good workout, feels great, repeats, gets into better shape, then feels even better. A KABOOMER has attitude and energy to handle stress and fix problems, and then gainfully gets on with enjoying life. Exercise-generated *endorphins* improve your mood and make you feel better. When your mood is sunny, you can frolic, and you can keep from sweating the small stuff. Ninety-five percent of life is small stuff—right?

An angry flash of the obvious is shown in this NICABM Infographic (below):

- **Anger** adversely impacts our noggin, drives our hormonal system loco, and our heart, gut, immune system and pillow pleasures suffer.

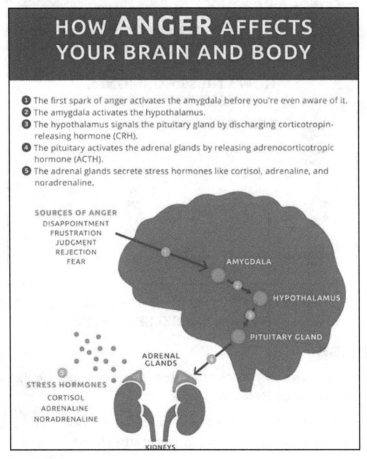

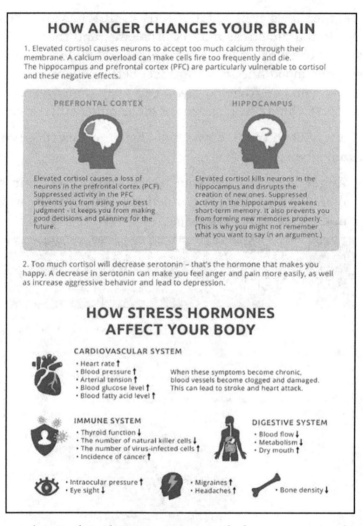

A movie-star/starlet acronym can help us counter bodily effects of stress. Try to be like CELEBS are. Be happy.

CELEBS

Try these *6 carefree hacks* to catch your life thief. Be like one of those carefree Hollywood celebrities.

1. **C**huckle. "Learn what is to be taken seriously and laugh at the rest." *Steppenwolf*, Hermann Hesse

2. **E**xercise to sweat (to release endorphin messengers). (See our *Stamina* and *Strength* chapters.)
3. **L**ove (to release special and pleasurable endorphins). Remember those good ol' B.T.O. lyrics about doin' it until...?
4. **E**at and drink well (to metabolize antioxidant plant foods, flavonoids, polyphenols, resveratrol from noble grapes). Be merry, too.
5. **B**reathe. Ripley would ask you to believe this or not:
   When you burn a pound of body fat, you exhale harmless gasses that have the same volume as a good-sized swimming pool. Believe it! Honest, folks. That CO_2 gives our planet's green plants half of what they need for photosynthesis and for life. (The essential other half is water.) Breathing deeply is a very fine practice with very big and healthy effects for de-stressing and sleeping soundly. The more you treat your pulmonary tissue as a responsive muscle, the longer you may live. Especially in pandemics!

My Grandfather, a Vermont country doctor, called pneumonia an "old gentleman's friend" for elderly patients. Hmmm—I'm not so sure I want that *friend* in later years, as I already had it twice in my mid-life. I acquired a very nasty mycoplasm pneumonia—just after Muppeteer Jim Henson died from a similar pneumonia. When we got ahead of it, my doctor said that my good protoplasm helped my battle. Breathe, folks! Even if you contract a bacterial or viral lung condition, deep breathing should help you as it helps me. Be your own best ventilator.

I carefully monitor my client's breathing prowess for exertion and stress indicators. Breathe, because oxygen is tantamount to life.

6. **S**leep. Grandma was right—you shouldn't go to bed angry, but you should go to bed early enough at about the same time to gain rest and lose calories. Yup!

Our brains are both amazing and strange. A big percentage of most boomers' daily calorie burn occurs *when* they sleep. Z's are our system reboots—yes? And when you are rebooted and refresh, steps are springier, loads are lighter. Mindful fun is habit forming. "Sleep serves to reenergize the body's cells, clear waste from the brain, and support learning and memory. It even plays vital roles in regulating mood, appetite and libido.... Sleeping is an integral part of our life, and as research shows, it is incredibly complex.[95]

However complex, those hours of pillow time are good for you—for improved mood, appetite, and libido. Sleep well and long. And be habitually grateful each night for another day of delight on this planet, among friends, and anticipating stamininety. When you do, you are guarding your physical 401(k) wallet and bank account from larceny.

Factor these six anti-stress steps, these six hacks, into your journey. In my book and yours, **KABOOMERs** are *CELEBS!*

When We Can't Avoid, Mitigate

If, and when life happens and stress is unavoidable—what can you and I do daily to *mitigate* it? A dozen upbeat hacks are offered as mitigation measures... **Avoid or Mitigate Your Stresses of Life**

1. Go ahead—enjoy that fidget spinner on your own or with a grandchild.
2. Take a walk in the woods and play Thoreau.
3. Break a sweat.
4. Master that word jumbler or Sudoku puzzle.
5. Laugh at "DC" Beltway shenanigans rather than fume about them. I listen to the Capitol Steps to help me in this regard.
6. Play with Fido or Felix the Cat.
   a. Laugh at your potty-mouthed myna bird.

7. Play rope-a-dope to dodge incoming hassles and use the ropes to bounce back.
8. Inhale, and breathe out slowly.
9. Zone out and "do nothing" when *nothing truly needs to be done.*
10. Don't internalize and fume; it is okay to let it out with a best friend or mate.
    a. Find a shoulder to lean on and arms to give you a bear hug.
11. If/when the SUCK truly arrives—take the #$%^ sandwich you're facing one day at a time.
12. A preacher once admonished that it was okay for me to curse, yet I should *never* blame. Good point, Reverend. Get past blame or fault and live.

Bottom line? Remember Hans Selye! Leverage your healthy habits to mitigate unhealthy stress levels. Develop and sustain yours, addressing these puzzle pieces to offset stress thievery 1. Soothing healthy food, 2. Exercise, 3. Restorative sleep, and 4. mindful relaxation surrounding your happy heart:

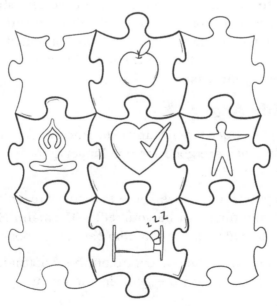

A healthy habit may take a period of *three to six weeks* to become ingrained. Also, some "mental" habits take longer to become ingrained in our grey "muscle memory." Duh...your stamininety prospects are higher when you adopt and sustain healthy habits—habits to manage stress actions and your reactions. *Twenty-one days* isn't forever. Breathe a little deeper. Count backward from 100 by 7's, laugh often, chase Fido, be playful, be one of the chosen CELEBS. Or, as author Mark Mason advised in his colorfully titled book, master "the subtle art of not giving a f*ck."

Attitude and Gratitude

Do cute little penguins or dolphins get angry, or hold grudges against their Dilbert bosses? Think about that. I'll bet a Koaching session that it is hard to be angry when you gaze at one of 'em or see Dr. Patch Adams in action. And it is a simple truth that you cannot be angry *if* you are grateful. *Gratitude* is important to our KABOOMER beings and our de-stress efforts.

Example: We can be subsumed by our aged parent's declines in health and mental acuity, or we can shift our life skill vantage to one of gratitude for their procreation and love (hopefully). Or, you lose a loved one, as columnist Chris Erksine did; and then celebrate the good times you had as time slowly eases your loss.

Set Aside Anger

Bad things happen when thing gets stuck in our craws. None of these baddies are good for our longevity or quality of life. Be still and mindful.

"Within you is a stillness and a sanctuary to which you can retreat at any time and be yourself."—Hermann Hesse (*Note that this quote is from the guy who penned* Steppenwolf*?!)*

Retreat to your happy place, up on the roof (thanks, James Taylor), in fresh air, in the gym, in the forest, by the ocean.

Wherever it is—gain that mindful stillness—to be your best KABOOMER self.

Breathe by BOXing!

If you can count to the number four, you can follow these four "boxed" steps to de-stress, as Uncle Sam's special warriors do. Your heart rate should lower as your distress drops, whatever life tosses you (whether it is a hand grenade or a lousy checkout clerk). One, two, three, four...

- Inhale for 4 seconds
- Hold for 4 seconds
- Exhale for 4 seconds
- Hold for 4 seconds

Do this 4 times, and you will lower your respiration rate, heart rate, and cortisol pump, I assure you. Do try.[96] A minute very well invested. Well, a minute and 4 seconds...

Yes, there are variations for the same inhale-hold-exhale process cited in the BOX method, perhaps a four-seven-eight second sequence.

Use Dr. Google to find other mindful breathing strategies—then practice, practice, practice. You'll easily locate motivational guru Tony Robbins for his chosen way.[97] Quickly get past anxiety and stress (in any season)—breathe it, feel it and get that heartfelt gratitude going.

Find the Light!

Lighten-up tips to manage stress are:

1. **Let It Go**
   Chill out (as sung by Idina Menzel in the movie *Frozen*).

2. **Tune In, or Out**
   Some relaxing musical genres are classic relaxation.[98] This doesn't mean loud Led Zeppelin before bedtime, duh.

3. **Say Sayonara (or Adios or Au Revoir or Aloha) to Stress**

A self-realized and self-actualized boomer can use his/her empathy and social skills to walk away or face-down a stressful situation. What's your emotional intelligence (EI)? Follow EI expert Dan Goleman or watch some top TED Talks[99] to learn more about EI. You too can say Adios to extended distress.

4. **Relax**

    Granted, this can be easier said than done on our treadmill of life. Say after me: this little hassle isn't worth cortisol's after-effects. Do you really need to experience America's Public Enemy Number One, as described by *Psychology Today*?[100]

5. **Have a Merry Heart**

    Do the following, as the good Doctor Patch Adams (pictured below) prescribes, to increase your *immunity*:

Chuckle. Socialize. Get fresh air. Walk barefoot. Exercise.

A Koaching note. I met that colorful and whimsical Doctor Patch late one night at Logan Airport. Gotta love that guy who makes patients' hearts merry!

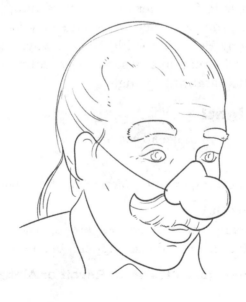

Or, think about a scripture verse:

"A merry heart doeth *good like a medicine*: but a broken spirit drieth the bones."—Proverbs 17:22

Do not let broken spirits into your physical bank!

Take note: Be merry, relax, eat properly, and exercise to beat lingering distress. If stressors in your day want to make you scream, break a sweat! Yes! A little exercise can make a big difference in your day.

Work out to counter stress and boost your thyroid function. Cardiovascular, strength, and flexibility exercises are all good ways to shape up *and to de-stress. Why? When you exercise, your body releases feel-good hormones, like endorphins, which can put you in a good mood. Remember, you won't die from sweat but you may die early from extended stress.*

6. **Smiles Beat Stress**

   Both our heart and brain benefit from hearty chuckles - not - smirks or scowls. One University of Maryland cardiologist, Michael Miller, suggested that laughter may be as good for our arteries as is aerobic activity. Please don't think that you need to emulate Jay Leno or Marvelous Mrs. Maisel as a standup comedian. Just give it a go. Laugh at your bad joke or pun but deliver it!

Dr. Miller offers a simple smiley prescription that won't bankrupt you and could save your life: "Thirty minutes of exercise three times a week, and *15 minutes of laughter on a daily basis* is probably good for the vascular system," he says.

Hee Haw

Try to laugh on a regular basis, as in *many* times each day. If anyone asks why you are joking around, just respond that "joking is good for my endothelium and longevity." That oughta shut them up. Or better yet, make him or her chuckle too!

The result of laughter is *priceless* for longevity and wellness:

- It reduces pain and allows us to tolerate discomfort.
- It reduces blood sugar levels, increasing our glucose tolerance—a very good thing.
- It improves our job performance, especially if our work depends on *creativity and solving complex problems*.

Its role in intimate relationships is muy importante—right?

In full agreement with Dr. Miller and Dr. Patch Adams, Deepak Chopra underscores laughter's role as good medicine. Read on for his half a dozen reasons to grin, chuckle and joke (even if you're not quite comical). If you are hesitant to trust my humor, trust him: chopra.com/articles/6-reasons-why-laughter-is-the-best-medicine.

Why Laughing Is Good Medicine

1. **Laughter Is Contagious**
   The discovery of mirror neurons—what causes you to smile when someone smiles at you—gives credence to the belief that laughter is contagious.

2. **Laughter Reduces Stress Responses**
   When you laugh, there's a contraction of muscles, which *increases blood flow and oxygenation*. Resultant releases of endorphins help you relax, physically and emotionally.

3. **It Boosts Your Immunity**
   According to one study done at the Indiana State School of nursing, mirthful laughter may increase our white blood cells that attack cancer cells. I like that!

4. **Laughing Increases Your Resilience**
   People who are resilient are happier and more successful. Laughing at mistakes allows us to recognize that making errors is a part of being human. This is indeed proof positive that I am human. Yeah!

5. **It Addresses Depression (Chemically)**
   Laughter releases a cocktail of hormones, neuropep-tides, and dopamine that can contribute to improving your mood.

6. **Laughter Relieves Pain (honest!)**
   People who laugh report that they are less bothered by pain experienced. It's not about changing pain levels. Laughter by itself isn't the solution, yet it can help a person *overcome* discomfort.

Thank you, Deepak. Now, what about food, and our "pri-mal" feeding? Don't get in a frenzy!

Diet to Douse Stress

Don't be or become an emotional or comfort food eater, please. Do try anti-inflammatory foods, many from the ground, which I group in the nutrient category of Vitamin *P(lants)*. Other stress-dousing nutrients from our seas (namely oily fish such as sardines in your Caesar Salad and yummy wild salmon as your entree). Anti-inflammatory foods *counter* stress! Keep emotions in check. Why?

Emotional eating is real. Been there, done that, in my days of yore. Perhaps you or someone close to you has unfortu-nately also been there, done that. Emotional and comfort eat-ing is not a healthy routine. Honest. Eat to live, and to enjoy your slowly chewed and tasty nutrients to douse stress, even if you're looking after one in the Greatest Generation, as my wife and I are.

Coping as Caregiver

How about those many of us who are caregivers to our elders?

Question: Did you know that we Medicare-aged folks have our very own **Institute of Stress**? I kid you not: www.stress. org/seniors.

Please reflect on the numbers that count from that seniors' stress site:

"Seniors who felt stressed out from taking care of their disabled spouses were *63 percent* more likely to die within four years than caregivers without this form of stress. In another study...(adult) children who provided such constant care shortened their lives by as much as *four to eight years*. Caregivers also had double the rate of severe depression...and this can increase risk of death by as much as *four times* when compared with non-depressed controls."

Ouch! Valuable tips to reduce caregiver stress, when you find yourself in those *un*enviable shoes, are:

Caregiver Stress relief
- Identify what you can and cannot change.
- Set realistic goals that you can do individually when you have time.
- Don't hesitate to ask for, and to accept, assistance.
- Don't be afraid to ask family members to contribute their fair share.
- Find and leverage one or more support groups.
- Try to find time to be physically active as much as possible, to get enough sleep, and to eat properly.
- Make time each week to do something that you enjoy and can look forward to.
- Go up on the roof, as James Taylor suggested, "when this old world is getting you down."

Don't worry, please. People who take an active, problem-solving approach to any caregiving issue are much less likely to feel stressed than those who react by worrying or feeling helpless. Caring for yourself?

Is It Really Time for Your Gold Watch?

As a mid-year group boomer (born in 1953), I confess that I am gladly *failing* retirement. The "Gig Economy" has been very, very good to me as I like motion, coaching, and contributing.

Retirement, for some, may be an unfortunate case where poor planning predicates p#$% poor performance. My mom used to say this when I missed her mark, leaving out the p#$% descriptor. Generally, I trust the *Wall Street Journal,* and the *Journal's* Encore reporters wrote an article on April 22, 2019, entitled "The Case Against Early Retirement." It depends what "early" retirement operationally means to you and yours.

The Journal's punch line?

- Don't leave your office "too soon" and don't retire at age 62 or 65 "because that is the way it's always been." *Some* early retirees have had quickened loss of cognition and diminished physical/emotional health as sadults. That's hopefully not the case for "big gulp" KABOOMERs.
- In this same Encore edition of 2019, reporter Glenn Ruffenach performed a lesson-learned for his own retirement from rat races. You might pick up a post-mortem (so to speak) pearl from Glenn's observations about coping with life after work:

  1. He found himself going in too many directions to achieve his golden year goals. Being stretched too thin, even for worthwhile volunteer causes, was stressful over time.
  2. His wife and he worked out their "married for much yet not for lunch" routines. They communicated effectively, most of the time.
  3. He tweaked his dynamic balance between "engagement and freedom." It is perfectly okay to say "no" to a worthy cause. What is that worthy cause gonna do—dock your pay? I think not!

There you have 'em, viable and valuable ways to counter stress thievery. Your stamininety goal is to party when you are ninety years young. Partying is so *counter-stress* for us who thrive and strive. You won't be the life of the party if you stressed yourself to an early epitaph. You will give those parties life when you are happy-go-lucky. Rise. be gritty. Don't inflame your gut, and don't go to bed angry. Get physical contact, guffaw, love your natural opioids, and breathe. As Leonard Nimoy advised, your physical 401(k) will live long and prosper with less stress. Yes, you can be resilient.

What about Morpheus and countering sleep zombies? Who wants to cheat death?

CHAPTER 7

Mimic Morpheus When You Sleep

"Sleep is the Swiss army knife of health. When sleep is deficient, there is sickness and disease. And when sleep is abundant, there is vitality and health."—Matthew Walker PhD, neuroscientist and sleep researcher, Author of *Why We Sleep*

A KABOOMER *can* convincingly cheat death, like the Greek god Morpheus. Or like the character Morpheus in *The Matrix*. Soak that in for a minute. You can *cheat death*, and gain a few extra years, with restful sleep (as your utility knife). This is our lone case for cheating. KABOOM.

The following is *not* a typographical error:

One-third of all boomers, both males and post-menopausal females, have diagnosed or undiagnosed sleep disorders! Some of these problems, like Obstructive Sleep Apnea (OSA) can be life-threatening. I confidently state that sleep disorders can be accommodated. Your Koach is living proof.

Proof Positive

Years ago, my wonderful wife timed my nighttime breath stoppages at 60-plus seconds. Back then, I also had trouble getting home on my 45-minute commutes without dozing. My breath stoppages, highway scares, and party doze-offs were tipping points to get medical help.

I didn't smoke (except for a celebratory Cubano). I didn't drink alcohol to excess. I'm wasn't overweight. My neck circumference was above average. Yet it was, and is, a lean neck. I am lucky that I never faced post-traumatic stress disorder (PTSD). None of these top causes of OSA were *my* causes. Rather, my relaxed soft palate triggered "moderate" OSA, and that *coulda* killed me. Honest.

I don my Darth Vader CPAP mask regularly to celebrate restful sleep and stay alive longer. CPAP is shorthand for a **C**ontinuous **P**ositive **A**irway **P**ressure system that chooses the right pressure to stimulate "regular," non-Apnea sleep.

I *jest* about my mask's look and feel. Technology upgrades offer us smaller, lighter, and less hassle masks and machines every year or two. Lots of folks give up on their sleep masks, yet they *shouldn't*. Get over any hassle, folks. It is your life and breath, after all. Perhaps consider surgery as your alternative step, but Do Not be like that River called De Nial.

Machine noise is preferable to high decibel disturbing snores, right? To be clear on that aspect, a snorer may *not* have apnea. Yet a person with apnea likely snores regularly, and often when his or her body reacts to lack of oxygen. I love my deep sleep and I am very partial to stayin' alive, stayin' alive. I love that my sleep is much better these days. My KABOOMER body processes can release my natural human growth hormones, restore my noggin's clear thinking, and promote muscular repair after my workouts and activity.[101]

Do *not* live in denial, avoiding professional help for something so precious as your Z's. Women may suffer OSA as much as men after menopause. Three (of many) more sleepless Facts of Life are:

1. Less sleep, less caloric burn for our basic metabolic rate.
2. Less sleep, less cleansing of our brain circuitry.
3. Less sleep, less stamina and strength to git it on and keep it on.

Let's agree on what sleep is, thanks to Webster, or to dictionary.com (but not its sexual relationship meaning—yet). Sleep is: "a naturally-occurring, reversible, periodic and recurring state in which consciousness and muscular activity is temporarily suspended or diminished, and responsiveness to outside stimuli is reduced.[102]"

Reality Check

Very *few* of us will sleep like a baby tonight, even if we say Morpheus. *Trivia*; morphine stems from that sleepy Greek figure's name. Wouldn't it be nice to sleep long and hard like that cherub; without a care in the world?

In our world, much is speed-racing through our minds. Healthcare matters of our Greatest Generation take their toll; most lady boomers endure exhausting hot flashes; the guardian in you is worried about your adult kids' careers and their little ones. You get restless legs or cramps. And....

Why, Why, 600 Times Why?

A respected sleep guru, Sara Gottfried, offers genetic sleep *imperatives*: "...did you know that sleep governs over 600 genes? These include weight loss genes ... and genes that predict your risk of Alzheimer's disease."

The National Institutes of Health reports that, "many tissues in our body have their own clocks. The system is complex, with central clock genes directing the body's rhythms, deciding which proteins are expressed in which tissues at different times of the day. When our biological clock is disrupted, it can cause sleep disorders and a host of other problems, including obesity, depression, heart disease, high blood pressure and diabetes. Researchers... have found a new link between a circadian clock gene called 'nocturnin' and obesity."

You and **I need seven** to eight hours of sleep per night to lose weight. Why? Inadequate sleep chemically raises levels of ghrelin, that darned hormone that makes you hungry. Intersected sleep and chemistry, right? Sleep and wellness interacting, RIGHT?

Our National Sleep Foundation addresses wonderful Whys for restful Z's. Do check for your bespoke eye-openers at: www.sleepfoundation.org/how-sleep-works/what-happens-when-you-sleep.

This chapter's capstone cloud summarizes critical success factors to consider, and then leverage, to gain better sleep. Better restorative sleep beats counting sheep or being drunk! Eighteen hours without sleep can approximate one's brain fog from blood alcohol nearing legal limits (0.05 %) for driving.

Sleep for Is Not Overrated!

This chapter's wordcloud rates *sleepy* nouns and verbs, plus adjectives and adverbs for our consideration.

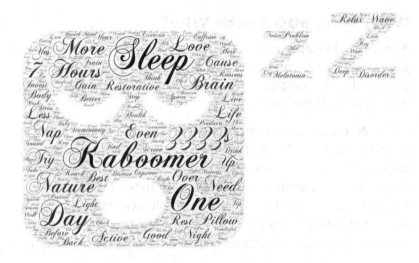

There are loads more scientifically proven reasons to get your restorative[103] sleep. And there are many, many methods that supposedly, possibly, or probably aid in your KA-BOOMER sleep. Trust, perhaps, yet verify. It depends what may work for you. Please avert what might be labeled insanity—doing the same sleep-deprived cycle repeatedly - while expecting better results. Please. Your help may even come from federally funded resources.

Hi, I'm from the Government and I'm Here to Help

Here are two federal "wake-up "calls:

1. "...a chronic lack of sleep increases your risk of obesity, diabetes, cardiovascular disease, and infections." [103]
2. "Because of your body's internal processes, you can't adapt to getting less sleep than your body needs." [104]

Please read that again! If your body needs sleep, you **cannot** adapt!

Your Guide to Healthy Sleep booklet **is** federal tax dollars put to good, preventative use.

As cardiovascular disease is the largest cause of illness and death for us Medicare-aged folks, I'm all aboard the Ben Franklin sleep train for worthy ounces of prevention. *How about you?* Sure, we sleep two hours less than Americans did a century ago. This guide also provides a fine summary of what our brains "do" while we are asleep. One hint: Our brains never take a break. Think about your own action steps to get quality time in deep, restorative sleep, please.

Poundage

We know that our brains are exercising heavily while we're in our nightly slumber stages. Well-documented studies record that our brains burn calories through our sleep time as much as 35- to 75-watt light bulbs would. *Wanna lose weight?* **Sleep!** If you have an average metabolic rate and sleep soundly for seven hours, that's about 450 dietary calories "brain-burned." That's correct. From one-quarter to one-third(!) of our "normal" daily caloric expenditures are sleep expenditures. And for good causes—like restoration, cleansing, and recovery.

Cleansing? Right. Our brains are fascinating in many ways. One fascinating fact is that our noggins do not have normal "plumbing" [lymphatic] systems like the rest of our bodies. If we don't sleep adequately, or exercise properly, [105] our brain's waste disposal system *cannot* complete its critical roles to keep us from exhaustion.

> "Insomnia! Devil
> that blends day into night and
> leaves us exhausted."—*A sleep haiku by
> Jenna Schneur, December 2012*

Sleep Zombies

Ever been sleep deprived? Likely happened more than once in your lifetime. Deprivation of restful sleep is *not* a good thing to sustain. Physical dangers or harm and certainly grouchiness will result from missed opportunities to restore and recharge your boomer mind and body.

Sure, we hear about individuals in Navy SEAL Hell Week, and other-worldly challenges, in which personnel can and do press on, like zombies. Ultra-endurance events, like extreme Mudder events, or the six-day, 140-mile trans-Sahara foot races, or those Badlands 135-mile ultramarathons (which start in Death Valley, California, each *July*), are very good for Guinness World Records.

Yet these overachieving participants experience *"Awful Afters"* as they face many weeks of recovery. And you could be living a lifetime of *"Awful Afters"* by being deprived of sleep on a nightly basis over years. You can't become or remain as a KABOOMER if you can't cope and mimic Morpheus.

Your Coping Capstone

Stamina is the bedrock for your journey to stamininety.

Strength activity is your cornerstone for vitality. Now...

Our **capstone** element of stamininety is...*sleep.* The capstone for putting years in your life and life in your years. *Isn't capstone a fine way to address your top "coping" and culminating achievements of your life well-lived and lengthened?*

What's in It for Me?

WIFM takeaways are your sleepy reminders and viable action steps.

- Restorative sleep is a critical part of your physical 401(k) account.
- Natural steps and products just may be fitting keys to our sleepy-ville door.
- Daily sleep of about seven hours is part of your recipe for respite.
- When you exercise, eat, when you get off screens, and how cool and dark your sleep quarters are can be 'lil bit extras for extraordinary sleep.
- Relaxation techniques and playmates do help.

Why Can't I Sleep? I'm Going Nuts

Our ability to sleep is tied to amino-acid conversion and neurotransmitter production of **serotonin**[106] and norepinephrine. Serotonin and norepinephrine are our natural, feel-good anti-depressants—and they are spell-check challenges too. Try to emulate the Beach Boys' good vibrations and elevate these key neurotransmitters!

What Causes Low Serotonin?

One medical professional, David Jockers (DrJockers.com), lists **Inadequate** or **Ineffective** Sleep as a *Top* cause for reduced feel-good vibes. As you've already read, there are inter-related causes and effects throughout our bodies and lives. Such is the case here for low serotonin! Six other limiters of our natural anti-depressants are:

1. Chronic/emotional stress
2. Poor sugar metabolism
3. Deficiency in magnesium*/vitamin A
4. Leaky (inflamed) gut
5. Inadequate omega-3 fatty acids
6. Deficiency in vitamins B1, B2, B6, and/or folate.

*Note: There are proven inter-relationships with one's feel-good chemicals and ingested nutrients. Magnesium (an essential micro-nutrient for many healthy matters) can aid and abet proper sleep, which can help keep serotonin higher.

• Low serotonin may also cause lower libido for women as, "some antidepressants can reduce one's sex drive. Your doctor might need to fiddle with finding the right medication for you. And they can take up to two months to work."[107] This known-unknown is of more than passing interest to many KABOOMER readers of both sexes. Now to another matter that can drive a sleep partner nuts—sleep disorders.

Sleep Apnea—Again

Apnea is a monumental sleep problem for millions of men *and* post-menopausal women. I'd be remiss if I didn't expand on this prevalent disorder which I cited earlier—from personal lessons.

America, we have a health problem. As one of approximately twenty million boomer sufferers, my own "sleepless in San Diego" journey may help some readers address theirs. Avoid trips on that unhealthy river "De Nial." I suggest that you check whether a loved one, or if *you,* have an unhealthy sleep disorder. Your sleep partner may already know if *you* do!

Don't let something which is correctible drive your partner and/or you batty!

If I was king, I'd regally prescribe a free sleep test for all. Priceless, proactive tests as positive impacts on your physical index funds.

More Sleep Thieves

There are other reasons for insomnia, or for one's getting up at night. I don't want these either:

- Restless Leg Syndrome (RLS), which is officially labeled RLS Willis-Ekbom Disease or RLS/WED these days— oy. I can and do get religious leg cramps after heavy weight-lifting routines, such as deadlifts and squats, but I have averted RLS thus far.
- Diuretics needed to address one's circulatory problems—ouch.
- Benign prostate enlargement (or worse)—a ya Chihuahua for us guys.
- Hot flashes for ladies—another *a ya Chihuahua* that sufferers do not take lightly.

Many ladies in our demographic, with their most unfortunate hot flashes, *can* be sleep-deprived. This I know from up-close and personal observations of my wife's sleep patterns and next day hypersomnia. It's *not* her fault.

If one or more of these *sleep thieves* sneak up on me, I will proactively pursue my restorative sleep; even if it means that I forego my *au naturel* philosophy. Sometimes, sleep is more vital than foregoing a short-term prescriptive pill.

Great Sleep as Capstone

Lights Out!

Get away from screens—smart phones, tablets, laptop computers—well before your *regular* bedtime. Don't watch ass-kicking war movies or intense sci-fi serials on any screen if it is late into your evening.

Kick ALAN in the glutes; that is, unless your bedmate is named Alan. (ALAN is an acronym for Artificial Light At Night.)

Your sleep partner (if present) and you should both avoid TV in the bedroom and also stop "blue" screen visits (e.g., tablets, laptops, smart phones, Kindles) *two or three hours* before bedtime. If you must finish a checklist for tomorrow, use yellow screen settings.

Nooners, Nappucinos, and Noise

Changing mindsets about napping at workplaces are pleasing to me. Midday "nooner" romps have long been the stuff of Harlequin novels and soaps—yes? Yet I'm more focused on naps as healthy midday activities. Yes, I nap on occasion. Before my late-night adjunct teaching, or after my before-dawn hours of power rowing on our Mission Bay, I will shut down to refresh and recharge. Yet I'm careful how to get this type of R&R.

Daniel Pink, our productivity pundit, offered (in *When: the Scientific Secrets of Perfect Timing*[109] and in his YouTube talk at youtube/UeXWQI8m_LM) when and how you or I can snooze effectively and efficiently.

(Dan's observations about best times to workout were offered in our KABOOMER Strength chapter.) *So, how about one's timing of 40 winks on any day of any week that ends in a letter "y"?*

Dan coined the term Nappucino[109] to brand this great nap hack, which works very nicely for me. Here's the hack: Drink your preferred caffeine beverage, hit the rocker or couch, or workplace desk, and tune out for a timed 20 minutes. Your caffeine boost begins in about that same 20 minutes. Splash some water on your happy mug and then restfully carry on with your day.

One's catch-up snoozes, or sleeping-in-later routines on weekends, holidays, or mental health days, **do** *address short-term sleep shortages* that are bad, bad in many, many ways. Who hasn't awakened refreshed after a 20-minute siesta? Put a little caffeinated zip in this equation and you are good to go. Note the approximate limit for a good nap—*veinte minutos* (20 minutes). Why? After a half-hour nap or more, you may have trouble shaking away your cognitive cobwebs, and this may impede that night's critical sleep.

Catch a Wave

Our active brains emit waves, which we now know we can emulate in order to relax and to ready our sleepy disposition.

The nonprofit Monroe Institute (with which I have no relationship) offers a provocative repository of noise signals to play, and techniques to use for enhanced sleep, consciousness, and self-awareness. I have acquaintances who swear by special, or white, noise to aid and abet their sleep. You might give some of these published techniques from Monroe or other sources a go.

This long Monroe weblink www.monroeinstitute.org/sites/default/files/Super%20Sleep%20%28Sample%29.mp3?uuid=5cbcaa45aac4a is a free 89-second sound bite of delta wave noise for "super sleep, which reportedly helps you produce the natural brain-wave patterns of the delta-sleep state; to enjoy the benefits of totally refreshing, deeply restorative sleep."

Here's another web source for your consideration regarding sounds for improved sleep habits: www.binauralbeatsfreak.com/brainwave-entrainment/9-things-you-should-know-about-delta-brain-waves.

Pillowing on, here is a great explanation of your nightly stages of brain activity pegged to wave signals: www.sixstepstosleep.com/sleep-stages-what-happens-when-you-sleep/.

This figure, offered by Six Steps to Sleep, may help you grasp healthy stages of your and my brain activity, day and night, while awake and asleep.

Brain Waves and Activity

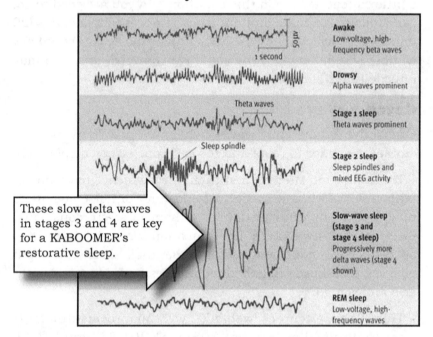

These slow delta waves in stages 3 and 4 are key for a KABOOMER's restorative sleep.

As shown, you need *deep* stage 3 and stage 4 sleep. You could listen to very low frequency delta waves before, and then during, sleep to dreamily count many sheep. Baaaa... I won't drill into Rapid Eye Movement (REM) sleep or other important matters for sleep in this tome. I'll save that for we-blog posts, my one-to-one Koaching sessions, or my practical Stamininety seminars.

Yes, you can find a multitude of relaxation sound applications in your smart phone App store(s). If you want to try sound for sleep-assists, here is what Inverse.com offers for its "top" seven applications.[110] Just use that phone of yours for relaxation—not text messaging or a few more emails—before your shut eye.

"Best" Phone Apps to Help You Fall Asleep

1. Noisli
2. Sleep Cycle Alarm Clock
3. Calm
4. White Noise
5. Pillow
6. Rain Rain Sleep Sounds
7. Stop, Breathe & Think.

Another reputable web source for online sleep applications is *Medical News Today.*[111] As with the Inverse citations, most of the downloadable sleep applications from *Medical News Today* are **free**.

What About You, Koach?

I've tried sounds of nature, and those were certainly relaxing for me. Falling asleep, however, is not my issue. As a Navy guy, shipboard life made me learn to get to sleep quickly. Rather, as I get older (not *old*, as I'm a KABOOMER), I find that I sometimes awaken after five to six hours of sleep. Whatever the root cause for my episodic stirring (sleep partner, temperature, leg cramp, a nightcap...), I can usually get back to sleep, and I appreciate that capacity. I acknowledge that others may not be so blessed as am I for restorative Z's.

Each of us has his or her own bespoke challenges and admirable sleep traits. My homily is that we should *all* strive to do better at something that is so precious and life-extending!

Yes, and How?

Dr. Gottfried shares trusted tips[112] for falling asleep quickly and to staying asleep, to gain health and beauty benefits from rapture in the deep.

Two micronutrients (stay tuned for more in your Clean Eating Chapter) that have a real say in your rested day after a blissful night are:

1. Vitamin D3 (naturally, if you can—with 20-minute exposure to our sun).
2. Magnesium absorbed over time via one's diet, vitamin supplement, or mineral baths. Why? Magnesium counters our stress response, and this good ol' micronutrient (when absorbed) helps our muscles relax.

Don't forget your and my second brain, *our microbiome (gut).* *Yup.* Our gut has a key role in our endocrine system's handling of serotonin (the happy hormone). I believe that my happy tummy directly relates to my happy and extended sleep pattern.[113] Do you?

Positions Please

If your mattress and pillow combination support side sleeping, you might try to sleep on your side (our right side is preferred, according to some experts, due to our heart's orientation). And you can always rearrange or add pillows to get yourself comfortable.

Do talk to a sleep professional about mattress and pillow firmness. Simple things like a crick in one's neck from too soft or too hard supports can monumentally mess with one's quality Z's.

Keep Cool

Night sweats and stress can disrupt sleep quality. Keep your room at about 64 degrees, cool enough to minimize hot flashes or night sweats. Wear something comfortable to sleep in. Enjoy your perfect pillows, and you might add one small pillow between your legs if you're sleeping on your side.

Limit Sleep Toxins: Alcohol and Caffeine

Half of all Americans have a slow metabolism gene for caffeine (as in many hours to absorb it). Thus, millions of us may become wired a few hours after our evening cuppas, turning into a sleepless mess. Alcohol causes similar problems for many of us, particularly if night caps are imbibed at closing times. Alcohol lifts cortisol, which may contribute to heart thumping awakenings in wee hours. Sure, some folks are luckier with their handling of caffeine and alcohol than are others. Some, like me, find that certain types of alcohol have wee-hour impacts that are greater than others. I also find, by the way, that summertime iced tea can wire me up more than my preferred social stimulant: coffee. Did you know that blonde or medium roast coffees may have higher caffeine concentrations than bold coffees? Check for yourself. Could you live with a diluted cuppa java, or drink de-caffeinated coffee, if you must have some in your normal evening hours? We also have exceptions to our routines, perhaps holidays or late evening airport pickups. In my case, teaching adult learners at night is an exception. I'm getting paid to be alert on my feet at 10 p.m., so I drink "leaded" coffee on my teaching nights. I'm blessed that I can generally fall asleep and remain that way after night teachings!

A Sleep and Stress sidebar

Female readers – you might consider taking this online hormone quiz from Dr. Gottfried at thehormonecurebook.com/quiz/take-the-quiz/. Guys – you can take this quiz too, but your results will likely be skewed.

Pillow Talk and Mattress Magic

Cervical pillows, oxygen pillows, apnea pillows: Buyer beware of much Madison Avenue hype about your own sleep train. Yet please don't rule out your pillows as enablers for spine stability, good breathing, and deep sleep.

And don't forget to find that ideal mattress that provides the best spinal alignment for your sleep partner (if applicable) and for you.

Should you want an eerie feeling, research how much of an "older" mattress weight is dust mites and their excreta. There are reasons to swap out that oldie pad and get a best possible mattress cover to keep mites out. These covers are worth your investment. My answer to the question posed in a *New York Times* article[114] is that I should be and am worried about household dust mites. Yuck.

Disclaimer: I am not marketing or endorsing products or services that are mentioned in my writing.

Habits

We are sleepers of habit; so my suggestion that you try a varied sleep position may go over like a lead balloon. I can only offer that I became a mixed back and side sleeper after my spinal fusion surgery. I was, until then, more of a regal snoozer and sleeper: face upward and flat on my back. I'm suggesting that by trying different positions, you might learn something and possibly get better sleep—particularly if you have acid reflux, back pain, snoring, apnea, or other relevant conditions.

Sleepwear or Not

In campfire days of my Eagle scouting, we sang:

> "And sometimes in the springtime and sometimes in the fall, I jump right between the sheets with nothing on at all."

Your scribe doesn't gain favor with nightgown and pajama dealers by suggesting you sleep with "nothing on at all." Yet health professionals and I can share healthy reasons why sleeping *without* PJs is good, or at least worth the proverbial try. Why not try it, if you haven't? You (and your human sleep partner?) may like it. And you just might be healthier too, even in fall and winter. I mentioned *human*, as there isn't a ton of research suggesting that a furry friend who shares your bed might enable your deep sleep.

Tim and I

Author and Podcaster Tim Ferriss offers interesting tips to unwind before his evening sleep: *Tools of Titans.*[115] Here is one:

- He invests 5-10 minutes to get his *To Do List* off his mind (which also drops his cortisol level a bit).

What have I tried to enhance restorative sleep, even when challenged by stresses and strains of my life?

Warm Epsom salt baths—finished 90 minutes before my lights out. We absorb magnesium through our skin pores, and actually "burn" a few calories when immersed and perspiring. My heart rate elevates, so I need some cool down time before calling it a night. Hence those 90 minutes between toweling and lights out. I find it both interesting and effective that a cool shower can have the same sleepy effect as that soothing bath, provided *that shower is finished* 60 to 90 minutes before you turn out your lights.

- My sleep professional once suggested that I try a prescription "lifeline" when I was pretty wired about a big workplace commitment. My MD suggested that I try putting one-half of a tiny Ambien tablet under my tongue if I couldn't sleep soundly till reveille. That seemed to work, and it was only used situationally.

- Note that I saw *a sleep professional.* Important things like sound sleep, for many reasons offered in this chapter, are best not left to rubes like me.

- Mellowing melatonin: Our "Paleo" forbears could generate plenty of natural melatonin and slept hours more than we do. After singing around the campfire and staring at the cosmos, there was a good argument to log 12 hours of sleep. The only reliable light they had was sunlight, so their circadian dark times enabled melatonin production—in buckets. Yes, evidence suggests that *el sol* does much to light up and lengthen our KABOOMER lives! Nowadays, cities that never dim (unless there is a blackout), and our screen times plus artificial lights, mess with our *natural* melatonin processes. I'll cut to the sleep chase for adults only.[116]

When I travel across time zones by air, or if I train quite hard on a given day, or if I think I might need a real sound night "in the hay," I might take a small (two to three milligram) "quality" melatonin pill 30 minutes before my intended sleep start. Two key operatives in my case: First, I don't mind this little mellowing ritual, as natural melatonin is within us (just like cholesterol production). Second, this is *as needed*—not as a nightly habit. No, I'm not fooled by the "natural equals safe" salesmanship we often see and hear in our screened digital lives. Trust yet verify, as President Reagan cautioned. Koach, what is your top travel hack? I have learned that best efforts to avoid time-zone zombie-ness is to be as rested as possible before starting my trip. Simple yet hard, I know.

Yes, world travelers may want or need prescription sleeping aids so that "jet lag" doesn't turn them into zombies. If so, I merely ask them to think about possible side effects of sleep aids, after *first* checking natural ways to get sleep for your time at 32,000 feet of altitude.

Our circadian rhythms normally elevate our melatonin level in the afternoon. Hence my, and possibly your, mid-afternoon slumps of energy and temporary drowsiness happen at about 3 p.m. local time. Grab twenty winks or a nappucino. Then get back to your refreshed KABOOMER day.

- **Is Red Wine mighty fine?**
  Yes, and no. Yes, to improve heart health, yet No for sipping as a sleep aid. Timing?! Despite antioxidant and mellowing aspects, nice red wines may cause you pre-dawn wakeups. Moderate your dinnertime and nightcap drinking. Sure, you should appreciate healthy anti-aging, anti-inflammatory resveratrol[117] in wines, but also appreciate that your "full" Z's may suffer. I find (unscientifically) that a jigger of "hard liquor" or spirits as my occasional dessert item doesn't seem to impact my sleep like red wine does. Nightcaps may help you get to sleep, yet generally

they will also cause you to stir and lose your deep sleep later.[118] In no way would I encourage a KABOOMER to start drinking for a personal sleep experiment. Live and learn.

Please try to form habits that help you gain those seven or more blissful hours on most nights! Shifting from drink to interesting food items . . .

- **Onions and Cupids?**

  These prebiotic[119] vegetables don't seem to promote my sleep, though some studies suggest the contrary. You might try this natural sleep aid (if you're sleeping alone, or perhaps if both your sleep partner and you eat 'em).

  I try to eat my evening meals early enough to get settled down. And not too spicy, being mindful of Satchel Paige's counsel. Not all onions are created equal – right?

  Koach, how about food which are labeled as "natural" aphrodisiacs?

  Yes, I say. Eat them to enjoy their taste and what nice consequences they may enable. You'll read more about love potions like chocolate, oysters, and strawberries in our Eat Clean segment.

- **Timed Exercise**

  Too late in the day for a good thing like exercise with elevated heart rates *isn't* wonderful. Morning times through early evening are the *best* times to elevate your heart rate with stamina or strength activity. For most of us, exercising too close to slumber times can defer or defeat our drowsiness. Why? Our excess post-exercise oxygen consumption (EPOC),[120] a.k.a. "afterburn", with elevated heart rate affects normal unwinding and pre-sleep efforts.

- **Sleep Potion**

  Tim Ferriss and others advocate this natural concoction to help with your nightly Capstone efforts:

  Mix organic apple cider vinegar with trusted-source bee honey and hot water. Sip, and sleep.

  Yes, the apple cider vinegar (ACV) taste takes a while to appreciate. Yet this pre-sleep drink may well provide a superior return on your investment. ACV is an historic, proven gut-helper too.

A Possible Sleep Problem— Over-training

Would you agree that sleep and exercise practices are integrated? I'll wager that you answered in the affirmative. See www.nfpt.com/blog/integrating-sleep-exercise-mutual-improvements.

Evidence

I have *never* heard an Olympic champion say that the real key to his or her gold medals was sleep-*deprivation*.

But I *did* read that the amazing Edwin Moses invested in 10 hours of restorative sleep daily for tip-top athletic performances. His 122-straight victories (No, 122 is not a typo) in grueling 400-meter hurdle events is amazing! I don't think I've ever slept 10 hours straight as an adult. And I'm certainly not "almost invincible"[121] as Moses was for nine years. Just sayin'....

Over-training impacts one's periodic rest and restoration as an awful after.[122] I love Mae West, yet I challenge her offering that "too much of a good thing is wonderful." Too much (and too often) exertion in our resistance activity can truly make us irritable, prone to illness, inflamed, and deprived of sleep. Your Koach has been there, done that. Not at all wonderful. It is great, I attest, to gain personal bests when you are training;

yet you may have a spouse whose own serotonin is also lowered by your fitful attempts to sleep. Trust your Koach; listen to your mind and body; and try not to over-train. Check?

Our sleep is very much *an active*—not passive—*process* of great value. You and I can count those valuable ways at http://sleep.org. Check this site, please.

Simple things, such as sleeping like a baby, can be hard. Yet managing stress (or distress) and gaining restorative sleep **will** help you thrive and strive into your 90s.

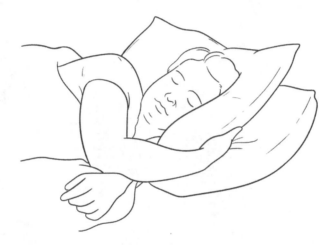

Onward, half a league onward with your sleepy capstone efforts! Enjoy your restful ROI. Those restorative Z's are a wonderful way to invest one-third of your life!

CHAPTER 8

Eat Clean, Age Slower

"It is curious *how seldom the all-importance of food is recognized.* You see statues everywhere to politicians, poets, bishops – but *none* to cooks or market gardeners."
— George Orwell, *The Road to Wigan Pier*

It is curious how often we hear of insta-diet improvements, gut-healing tricks, and overnight weight loss shenanigans based on exotic fruits or Old Testament lore or Hollywood doctor prescriptions. We've all heard countless dos and don'ts. Yet do not believe all that you read or hear. In my chubby youth, I heard that Wonder Bread was...wonderful...and that fat was evil. As an important point for this record, a wonderful war hero and public servant, Senator Jim McGovern, led a 1977 Congressional study that was (in my judgment) off the mark for healthy eating.[123]

"Undercooked science" about low-fat diets abounded then and persists to this day. TV dinners and processed foods were conveniently mass marketed as wholesome in my "not so happy" days. Wrong! My past was not a clean-eating past. And your earlier days may also have included "poor quality diets." That's a historic shame, if you recognize "the all-importance of food" as I now do. Here's an all-important math reality to recognize:

EAT WRONG = AGE FASTER and DIE EARLIER

Remember this: when you eat "wrong," your cellular damage accumulates *like a cancer.* You read that correctly; *like a cancer.* Wanna be wrong about this *all-important* matter? No!

Repeat after your Koach: I won't be wrong and increase my deadly risk. Shifting to right from wrong, I trust what the American Cancer Society offers for risk reduction,[124] as you should too:

"About 20 percent of all cancers diagnosed in the US are related to *body fatness, physical inactivity, excess alcohol consumption, and/or poor nutrition,* and thus could be prevented."

Say what? Twenty percent of *all* cancers *could* be prevented? This credible cause-and-effect statistic is very, very *wrong.* Many, many baby boomers *could* mitigate their body fat, move more, watch their alcohol consumption, and EAT CLEAN. Yet, millions (!!) of baby boomers blatantly **do not.** *That's what is wrong.*

Poor, unhealthy nutrition causes damage to our billions of cells each, and every day...if we let it. **Don't!**

Wrong Ways for baby boomers abound, due to Madison Avenue marketers; our corn economy zealots; fast food national trends; Wonder Bread; processed foods; saturated fats; nitrate-cured meats; char-blackened entrées; trans fats; high ratios of omega-6 to healthier omega-3 fatty acids; avoidance of colorful fruits and vegetables; eating big meals throughout the day; too many "simple" carbohydrates; sugar-rich "energy" bars; bad habits; etcetera, etcetera.

Let's consider poor nutrition and high body fat as causes of death for TV/movie star James Galdofini. *The Sopranos'* star passed from cardiac arrest in early 2013 at age 51.[125] His untimely demise curtailed my novice acting career. This is a personal play for me, and a reverse role-modeling message for you.

When serving as president of the San Diego Rowing Club, I received a surprise phone call. A jingle from a movie producer about a sports movie. A flick with my special sport, rowing, as part of the storyline. A storyline that commissioned *real* actors Christopher Lloyd and James Galdofini. We shot our cameo crew scenes on Mission Bay one morning and hoped for a big screen release. Well, the big screen never arrived. Our marquee lead, James Galdofini, passed away before his "shoots." That was my last $58.00-day as an aspiring actor, but that was far from my last day of rowing (thankfully).

Add Galdofini's "way of life" diet to his ample alcohol consumption, and what resulted? *Muerto.*

Your Koach asserts that a clean diet woulda coulda improved Galdofini's lifestyle and longevity.[126] So, what is our awesome alternative, here and now, *regardless* of one's current cardiovascular condition?

Eat clean to improve your chances to party past 90.

Eating clean equals eating quality nutrients, habitually. By eating clean, you slow damage and inflammation to the cells that make you who and what you are. I took many moons to learn right from wrong in this food context. My clients know that my dietary experiences can help them. Now, I intend to help *you.*

But first, *KABOOMER: Thriving and Striving into your 90s* is not a diet book. Or a Weight Watcher's book. I am not a registered dietitian, and I do not count calories. As habit, I eat adequate and healthy macronutrients and micronutrients, and I drink plenty of clean water. How and when I consume those life-saving nutrients is key to my daily habits. (By the way, my editors put my original unabridged chapter for Eat Clean on a *diet*. You were rescued from my overwriting).

But I will tell ya what, when and how you lessen your cellular damage with clean eating. How *slowly* do you want to age? Duh.... I commend to you these "eat right, fight aging" habits from author-athlete Matt Fitzgerald. Matt's six-step process can be added to your stepping for physical improvements, as I did.

Six Anti-aging Steps toward Stamininety (while offsetting Metabolic Syndrome*)

1. Fix your diet quality (for both macro- and micronutrients). *'Diet quality' is a synonym for clean eating.*
2. Manage your appetite (good fats and hydration help here).
3. Balance your energy sources (eat more than just meat and potatoes) to help offset metabolic syndrome.
4. Monitor your progress and process.
5. Time your ingestion of nutrients.
6. Train (move and breathe).

* **Note:** Metabolic Syndrome[127]—trust your Koach that the only good thing about this syndrome is its avoidance. Stay tuned for more about these unhealthy, clustered abnormalities.

Fix... Manage... Balance... Monitor... Time... Train.... Strive to KABOOM in six simple-sounding steps, starting with dietary habits.

Diet Quality

You'll know a high dietary standard when you experience it.[128] Honest. But first, a quick anecdote before we bite into your quality, diet-driven performance as a KABOOMER:

Japanese eat very little fat, drink very little red wine and suffer fewer heart attacks than Americans. The Mexicans eat a lot of fat and suffer fewer heart attacks than Americans. The French drink excessive amounts of red wine and suffer fewer heart attacks than Americans. The Germans drink a lot of beer and eat lots of sausages and fats and suffer fewer heart attacks than Americans.

Conclusion: Speaking English is apparently what kills you.[129]

I jest about the Queen's English. Yet I'm deadly serious about clean dietary habits and sustenance. Piling on, Dr. Michael Greger states: *"The number one cause of death in America is the American diet.* [130]Yikes. That's a number one you *don't* want to claim.

Make a deliberate detour around this *top* cause of mortality in our nation. Diet quality enables that detour. Trust Doc Greger and trust your Koach. Now, trust Karen Collier's guidance for diet quality.[131]

1. Include food choices and amounts...*to meet recommended goals and limits.*
2. Achieve and *maintain a healthy weight.*
3. Get a larger proportion of calories from *more healthful foods.*

Embrace these guides as starting points for your habitual *highs*:

1. Meet your goals with *right for me* choices and amounts.
2. Maintain a *right* weight.
3. Don't eat crap, as authors Crowley and Dodge advised in *Younger Next Year.*

Diet Quality = Eating Clean, regardless of your preferred diet or the source of macronutrients you consume. And regardless of what your *generalized* body type, or somatotype, is—whether skinny, middlin' or fatty. A quick breakout of those Greek words for three body types (devised by a psychologist in the 1940s):

a. "Skinny" folks who can eat blubber without gaining body mass are called **ecto**morphs. *Ecto* means "external" and *morph* means "form or structure." You can see evidence of an ectomorph's internal abs, muscles and vascular veins from external views. He or she may not have bulging muscles, but he or she has low body fat. Think of a distance cyclist or runner. Then think of a soccer player as an ectomorph. Life isn't perfect for older skinny minis. Why? Gaining muscular weight is hard, and frail physiques can be damaged easily.

b. Folks who are a bit stockier, who can lose weight, yet can also gain fatty weight, are called **meso**morphs. We think of football linebackers or tight ends, or most rowers, as mesomorphs. They (and I) are more muscular and heavier than those skinny ectomorphs who we sometimes like to dislike.

c. Plumper or portly folks who can't seem to shed their fatty poundage are called **endo**morphs. Marilyn Monroe might have been an endomorph, so this third category for body type ain't all bad in all respects. As an endomorph, a chubby couch potato can pack on pounds readily. This poundage (mostly around one's middle) may not be a personal packing fault, as genes and endocrinal glands **are** in play. Yet *unhealthy* fat is...unhealthy. You just read what Dr. Greger advised. Now heed that.

What's your approximate body type? Just askin'.

Muscle up > < Fat down. And stay tuned for a critical indicator for health & fitness for all three types called *Waist to Hip Ratio* (WtH for short).

Next, let's consider the types of nutrients we ingest by want or need.... What type of macronutrient eater/ devourer/swallower are you? Are you an omnivore like me? Or a carnivore? Possibly a herbivore? Chew on this word "*vore*" which means "devour or swallow." Speaking of devour, A guy named Bacon offered that some books should be devoured. Please devour KABOOMER!

Vore

You are an individual "vore", whether you speak Latin or not. You may eat both meats and plants as an *omnivore*. That's me too. You may eat only plants as an *herbivore*. I hope that you aren't a *carni*vore, as you'd miss many clean eating basics! Note: whether you do or do not eat meat, you can still KABOOM. Vegetarians can be strong and sustain their performance. A notable leading edge KABOOMER, Arnold Schwarzenegger, is now a "Terminator on a different diet" following his cardiac issues. Take his counsel to your own physical bank:

"There's this misperception that [animal protein] is the only way you get big and strong."[132]

Don't miss with your perceptions or actions! Speaking of this action hero–turned–state governor–turned–vegan, his six elements for success in life were offered to USC graduates in 2009:[133] *"Trust yourself, break some rules, don't be afraid to fail, ignore the naysayers, work like hell, and give something back."* Spoken like a true dinged yet enduring KABOOMER!

Trust yourself. Find, then stay with, what works for your clean dietary habit—what to eat, when to eat—and what quantity of vital nutrients do you need to eat to avoid the "apparent" perils of speaking English. **Note:** I didn't say *"Go on a fad diet."* Go to our enduring source for clean and quality nutrients called *sustenance*.

Endure, party, and prevail via sustenance; or "food and drink as *a source of strength and nourishment.*" *Sustinentia* means "endurance" habits.

And one more time: let's link our interrelated assets in our physical 401(k) account. Clean eating, as *physical currency,* improves a) bedrock stamina efforts; b) cornerstone strength thrusts to counter loss of muscle (among many other benefits); c) de-stressed and chilled demeanor; and d) restful, restorative sleep. *You are, indeed, what you eat.*

I'll offer this mighty metaphor as your clean dessert:

Your best way to showing great abs is through your refrigerator door!

Three nutrient classes that we need as physical currency are considered next. Then, let's add three plus one to consider four elephants that can squash us on our foody journeys to stamininety:

a. Unhealthy fat
b. Leaky gut
c. Metabolic syndrome and inflammation
d. Unclean and unhealthy dietary choices.

Four Elephants that Squash Stamininety

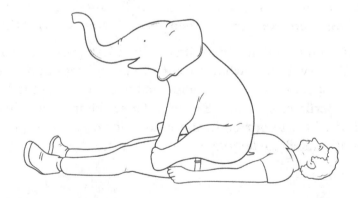

Should you be aware of these elephants that can sit on you? You betcha. Your Addenda are detailed segments at this book's end that you are entitled to skip. Just watch where these pachyderms are gonna sit.

Back to Stamininety diets....Know, or learn these *five certainties* to live long and to live well:

1. Most gains for stamininety stem from your *habitually healthy diet and drink.* We Master Fitness Trainers (with nutrition specialties) and coaches wish we were *tops* as critical success factors for clients' longer and better lives. Tops? Dietary habit and quality transcend impacts we trainers can have on folks like you. You *are* what you eat, to recycle that profound phrase.

2. Repeating for emphasis, your route to great "abs" is through your refrigerator door. And staying away from processed/packaged foods that don't spoil. Knowing when to eat, and how much nutrients we need to survive and thrive, are also good routing instructions! A shut door can be a very good thing, and your Koach can't close it for you.

3. Our ability to lose weight (fat) is first and foremost an *energy equation.* When we burn more energy (calories) than we ingest, we lose calories stored as body fat over time. Yes, there are hormonal and genetic factors at play for many boomers. I am living proof of that, as I have an inherited "fat" gene. Yet this energy equation still holds as the first principle for body composition for all three body types: Expend energy. Ingest less potential energy from your daily food or drink. Get leaner. KABOOM. Animals in almost every living species live longer when leaner. End of sermon.

4. An ounce of body fat prevention is worth far more than a pound of cure. Once white fat cells are generated by

our body, they dangerously persist in our aged midsections. KABOOMERs don't create more white fat cells. And they habitually shrink those persistent ones that they may have by eating cleanly and...wait for it...moving to sweat, as you know from your bedrock chapter of Stamina for Stayin' Alive. And moving stuff.

5. Diets, from their original Greek origin, are *ways of life.* And ways of life should be considered *habits. Pick good ones and stick with them at least 80 percent of the time.* Healthy habits that we practice become ingrained in our psyches and stomachs after about *21* days. Might be longer but won't be less than 21 days. I care not which clean dietary habits you sustain. Find a **way of life** that works for you. Yet hold this thought: *plant-based nutrients and low carbohydrates* are common denominators of most *leading diets* proclaimed by experts. DASH, Mediterranean, ketosis, and Paleolithic diets have common denominators: a. adequate quality proteins and fats; b. low measures of carbohydrates; and c. avoidance of simple, high glycemic sugars.

Note: These are *not* five easy pieces, yet these pieces *are* ageless truths that shape a KABOOMER's sustained journey to many parties past 90 years of age.

I could pen page after unabridged page of experiential and helpful details for you to consume, but I won't. Rather, I'll direct you to your Koach's online resources: wellpastforty.com and babykaboomers.com—and/or your nutritional experts. This is uber-important! *Eat clean to age slower.* Don't become a *reverse* role model who dies young. And find yourself a good role model or models. What About me?

Your Koach's Clean Eating Rubric

1. I will be patient, yet vigilant. I know that favorable changes to my body composition triggered by clean

eating will take time, possibly months. I will need *weeks* of good habits to see noticeable differences. I will *not* gain the boomer average of two pounds of fat over any year's winter holiday.

2. I won't worry about body mass or weight by itself. I don't count calories, though I do skeptically scan food labels and menus, and I keep processed foods at arm's length. However, I don't want to live like a prisoner of war or a monk. Food is first and foremost *fuel,* and fuel drives my energy equation for expending and ingesting calories as I KABOOM.

3. This one is tough to do yet important! I will ingest adequate protein—ingesting as much as possible or practical from plant sources. I strive for daily ingestion of three-quarters to one gram of complete protein for each of my 208 pounds. Note that this goal is above our government's suggestion, or the minimum daily requirement.[134]

4. I limit my carbohydrates; especially high glycemic index (GI) or simple sugars like fructose. I run and hide if I hear the four-letter word "HFCS." As a male KABOOM-ER, I use 100 grams daily as my "guy's" carbohydrate goal. (Fifty total grams of carbs daily is a good body composition goal for lady KABOOMERs). Yes – you can meet this daily goal as I do. *Remember that if you don't expend energy, those sugars end up as white, inactive fat.* Yuck.

5. I eat healthy fats! As a guy, I shoot for one-half gram of healthy fats and oils per pound of my body weight daily. (Ladies, do likewise for one-half gram of healthy fat per pound of your current body weight!) I enjoy healthy fats like avocados, wild salmon, and nuts as essential elements in my clean, balanced macro and micro pit stops! KABOOM. Yes: some nuts, like cashews,

can cause allergic reactions in me. If you're like me, be conscious of food sensitivities and find alternate sources of fat and fiber.

6. I drink water, as H_2O is a critical part of my healthy sustenance and muscle mass. I keep a non-plastic water bottle with me continually. I spritz my water with lemon for taste and as an anti-inflammatory boost. I add apple cider vinegar to my pre-breakfast hydro boost with lemon.

7. I count circumferences more than my poundage, knowing that my muscle is denser than fat. I will use my mirrors, the compliments of family members and friends, love-handle pinches, or body fat caliper measures, as my dietary and body mass feedback. How my clothes fit (slightly snugger tops for back, chest, neck, and shoulder gains, plus looser waists) is powerful feedback for body composition. *Have you heard the adage that kids, Lululemon leggings, and drunks are also candid indicators of body composition?*

8. I weigh myself once a week, on the same day, at the same time of day. I monitor my blood glucose levels 1 or 2 times each year.

9. I use a wrist cuff monitor for my blood pressure (BP) checks. I check my BP at home regularly. If my BP seems higher or lower than my "norm," I look for root causes and remediation, which can be related to food. (As a Koaching aside: I see an MD regularly, and I don't forego flu or hepatitis shots or pneumonia boosters.)

10. I monitor my resting heart rate daily. Caveat: a fitness watch or application *doesn't* ensure that you will get leaner or fitter! Honest. You may or may not need a fitness watch or smart phone application to measure your heart rate or to monitor calories. Our diet quality affects healthy heart function. Period.

11. I acknowledge body composition plateaus of little or no progress. I accept that there will be one of those plateaus at some point. I research ways to regain my progress. I adapt my energy equation and dietary habits, if stuck in neutral, to regain progress on my lean, long and well life's journey.

12. I recite my mantra that *"Great KABOOMER abs come from my clean diet and through my refrigerator door!"* I acknowledge that exercise regimens and activity have a minority share in my overall physical 401(k) account! I take **mesomorph** steps to wake up my chemical messengers for fat-burning and put to sleep my fat storage triggers.

There you have 'em: Koach Dave's dozen dietary hacks. My simple yet hard ingredients for a long recipe of thriving and striving.

What about Fasting and Intermittent Fasting?

I don't specifically mention intermittent fasting in these 12 testaments. Again, *KABOOMER* isn't a diet-specific book. I acknowledge that going without macronutrients for at least 14 straight hours in 24-hour periods can support clean living. I occasionally fast so that my body relearns how it can tap fat storage for my daily energy equation. Yet, I don't fast when intensity-based stamina or resistance training is on my periodized regimen.

What about you, dear reader? You read what works for me. Now, what about you? Your quality principles to eat cleanly? *What's in "it"* (meaning clean eating) for you? Here goes...

- Yes! Clean KABOOMER diets can *decelerate* inevitable aging. We must (by definition) get *older* to reach stamininety. Yet we should *not* get old. There is a *new* scientific field to examine "geroprotector" compounds that may indeed slow our aging process. Hold that big word and that tempting thought: *geroprotection*! Keep your ear to the ground to learn if turmeric's curcumin, red wine's resveratrol, and many other natural compounds serve us well when it comes to geroprotection and our anti-aging diet. I know what I intend to do; and I will keep my Medicare-aged ear open to new developments.

- Eat healthy fat. This somewhat counter-intuitive challenge is a requisite for *klean* KABOOMER nutrition, *great* fitness, and longevity. Get most of your healthy fats from plants and trees—not from meat sources or processed food in boxes! Note: meats *do* have needed fatty acids, yet your Koach's message to omnivores is to moderate, moderate.
- KABOOMER dietary habits favorably impact restful sleep, bodyweight, and workout performance (by day and night, between weight sets and between the sheets).
- Limit daily carbohydrate intake and further limit intake of "simple," high glycemic index (GI) carbohydrates as regular habits. As healthy fiber is classed as a carbohydrate "macronutrient," your other "GI"—your gastrointestinal tract—craves adequate quality carbs. Yup.
- Verify what clean dietary habits work best for you!

Online "help" that informally cites diet success of young Hollywood stars or America's biggest losers may *not* work for you. In my line of work, I am clobbered by daily *advice* for instant weight or waist loss with a magic elixir, carefree detoxification, and too-good-to-be-true panaceas. Do your research, then safely experiment with what works for your individualized journey. KABOOM. Significant dietary drivers are shown in this chapter's wordcloud below:

Significant Dietary Drivers for KABOOMERs

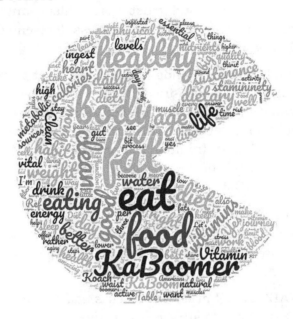

How?

When you ingest a solid or liquid that **_nourishes and sustains the critical needs of your body_**...you eat clean. I fully agree with Mayo Clinic experts[135] regarding these four healthy how-to habits:

1. Eat real food (and *skip* refined and processed convenient items).
2. Enjoy home cooking which beats Golden Arch convenience food for six of seven days each week in your journey. It's about your *nourishment*, not your convenience.
3. Go for plant-based foods if you want your best chance to be a centenarian. Spell after your Koach: *beans*. Honest, legumes are key to the lifespan of centenarians in Blue Zones.
4. "Clean up your act." Be active, get enough sleep, and manage your stress in healthy ways. Connect with people

you enjoy. Talk, laugh, share a meal, go for a walk, or play a game. Clean eating improves these already good acts—trust me. And trust that athletic author, Matt Fitzgerald, whose six-step process (presented earlier) will improve your physical 401(k).

Your family and/or friends may eat red meat every day, or eat regular plates of deep-fried chicken and gravy, or drink a lot of alcohol. KABOOMERs are big girls and boys who can break tradition to eat *good* nutrients. Remember these hacks: a) Avoid bad dietary traditions of *reverse role models* so you can party past 90. b) Sustain these three good nutrients in your life. KABOOM.

One, Two, Three

1. Macros are big. Size does matters, surely. *Macronutrients* are those biggest sustenance elements that keep us vital.

2. A KABOOMER must also seek *small* or *micro*-elements of sustenance to survive and thrive, to live long and live well. Our billions of body cells habitually need tiny vitamins and minerals that come (predominantly) from plant sources, our micronutrient source of *Vitamin-P(lant)*.

3. Our third component category of clean eating...is cool, clear and clean *water*.

Let's next review benefits of eating clean macronutrients and micronutrients and *drinking water before thirst.*

Eating clean six days a week and drinking vital H_2O every day each week unless you are a camel. Yes, I know that six is less than the Beatles' Eight Days a Week. (By the way, I rate both Sir Paul McCartney and Ringo Starr as KABOOMERs.) Take note, please: Experts write, and I agree, that successful KABOOMER journeys include a couple of meal hiatuses or day-trip excursions from strict clean eating. An implicit lifestyle rule is this:

Don't go *overboard or crazy* with overly strict habits.

That small portion of decadent dessert, or a few fried sweet potatoes with skins, or seconds at your Thanksgiving feast, won't detract from, and may *benefit* your sustained sustenance and livelihood. I know that sounds ironic, 'tis true. That six days a week pattern or the habit of eating *clean* is sometimes called "80/20." If your Koach can hit and sustain his clean 80/20 eating habit, you can too! *And* you can enjoy a treat without guilt. I know what's on your mind....

How Much is Enough?

Answer: *It depends* for macros, micros, and water on your body type, your innate metabolism, your stamina and resistance efforts, prescription drugs taken, your hormonal function, your sleep, and your stress patterns. This response is not a cop-out. How much you *need* today is likely different than the amounts you needed a decade ago. How much you *need* a decade from now may be different from today. It truly depends.

Take one macronutrient to its upper limit: if you eat or drink more than four grams of protein per pound of your current body weight, your kidneys will say no more! Duh, don't do that! Yet <u>do</u> ingest and absorb adequate protein to remain vital for many, many moons.

You need all *three* clean nutrient classes to live long and well.

What is this Koach's conviction, without meeting each of to learn of your bespoke "dependencies" for clean eating? (I hope that I will one day.) You likely need to eat clean quantities of macronutrients that exceed our government's recommended daily "recommendations." That isn't blasphemy, it is my experiential heady conviction. You possibly need supplements of select micronutrients that you don't get from food, or don't effectively absorb from the natural foods you eat. Let us also take an example of micros to the limit. If you lack adequate vitamin C, you can get sick, acquire scurvy, experience fatigue, and have sore gums, joint pain(s), poor wound healing, and even corkscrew hair. What KABOOMER wants those results of malnutrition? Satisfy your nutrient needs by counting uno, two, three....

I. Macronutrients

We *must* ingest enough macronutrients to support our primal 4Fs. Recall that those Fs are *fight, flight, feed, and frolic(sex)*. Macronutrients come in three variants: 1. Proteins (meaning *complete* amino acids); 2. Carbohydrates (which include healthy fiber); and 3. Fats. Yes, fats!

Your ingested amount and percentage of each macronutrient should vary based on your activity. Variances may also be necessitated by physical/mental conditions and doctors' orders. This shapes your basic metabolic rate and predicates muscle gain or fat loss each day, every day.

Example: a marathon runner from East Africa loads daily carbohydrates to fuel his or her long-distance running. Alternatively, one who is interested in averting sarcopenia (loss of flesh) will do his or her best to ingest and absorb adequate protein daily. Plus, protein absorption increases your metabolic rate, burning non-exercise calories. Plus, bigger and thicker muscles support your skeleton and help you avert falling, plus...you get my thought train. When you balance your macros eaten or drunk each day with your resting and active life, you should maintain your healthy weight (and fat level). Your physical performance under any circumstance, and hopefully your love life get big boosts too. A macro is a really *big* show, as Ed Sullivan used to say.

Macronutrients Fuel You

Macronutrients are simply yet importantly what KABOOMER bodies need in *large* amounts. That stated, we're talking about *grams* of "large"—rather than kilograms of "large." These nourishments provide our bodies with potential energy (calories):

1. **Fat**, our most efficient macro source of potential energy, provides or stores nine dietary calories per each gram eaten or drunk;

2. **Carbohydrate**, as our primary fuel for bodily cells (and why we should eat small amounts of *good* carbs), provides or stores four calories per each gram that you ingest; and

3. **Protein**, a least desirable energy source, yet a most important building block for skeletal muscles, also stores four dietary calories or KCAL per each gram ingested.

We need proper amounts of each macronutrient, yes?! Let's discuss how to go and get 'em.

Food, glorious food

"You are *what* you eat eats."—Michael Pollan, *In Defense of Food: An Eater's Manifesto*

We eat plants, directly or indirectly. We eat plants that magically processed sunlight and carbon dioxide to produce our food: Biochem 101. *What we eat* previously ate plants or ate something that ate plants. With one exception, that is. *Fungi*...You can and should eat certain fungi (which are not in the scientific plant "kingdom"), such as immunity-boosting shiitake mushrooms.

I'm a proud omnivore, though Michael Pollan wrote that I still have a "dilemma." (*The Omnivore's Dilemma* is another book I recommend that you devour, as R. Bacon suggested.) I reckon it is my prerogative at the top of our eats chain to healthily consume both plant-based and "hoof-based" nutrients. I have no problem at all with others' seasonal or permanent choices to eschew meat, eggs, dairy, or other "macro" food sources. It depends, yet again. Comedian Scott Adams offered this chuckle:

> "You're thinking I'm one of those wise-ass California vegetarians who is going to tell you that eating a few strips of bacon is bad for your health. I'm not."

Don't classify me as a wiseass or confuse me with a wise man. Rather, I offer that a few lean strips of *uncured* bacon may be good for health and testosterone or "T" factor gains for both men and women of our generation. Take that, Scott. Yet, thank you, Scott, as your healthy humor indeed reduces stress. Ha.

My meal preparations and most of my meals are part of my very good life and journey to party past 90. I *don't* live to eat gluttonously. Yet I surely enjoy cooking and eating balanced healthy meals, about 80 percent of the time (or five to six days out of seven days most weeks). Our 80/20 "habit—as diet" guideline is sustainable, healthy, and satisfying. A personal example: If I go astray for a bounteous holiday feast, I get back on to healthy habits the next day and stay with them until a next planned excursion. Does author Pollan highlight bad boys that may contribute to our societal problems of obesity and adult diabetes? Indeed.

He hammers *corn*. Not corn as a wholesome source of some micronutrients. He chastises our sugary, "super-size it" economy built on corn. Please don't get me started on the dastardly evils of high-fructose corn syrup [HFCS]. Repeat after me: high glycemic index (GI) carbohydrates such as HFCS are *bad, bad* choices for my healthy, proportional carbohydrates. Bad by a very long shot! And I won't get started on "GMO" here.

Don't get me on a roll either about our sad *Fast Food Nation*. This non-fiction epic published in 2001 by author Eric Schlosser tells how it was (and is) for folks in a nation which to this day consumes convenient *junk*. Golden Arches,

Kentucky Fried Chicken, and Taco Bell—*peligro*! Processed food=a definite skull and crossbones!

Schlosser contends that fast food "has altered the landscape of America...fueled an epidemic of obesity and transformed food production." *Major league "Oy"!* Note that I didn't add *for the better* after that transformation quote. What macro-food *does* transform us for the better? **Beans**.

Beans and legumes are *so fine* as age-arrestors and inflammation-fighters. Yup. The author of *Blue Zones,* Dan Buettner, offers "Beans" as a *most* significant factor for centenarians' health and longevity. Buettner's excellent TED talk is called "How to Live to Be 100."[136] Macronutrients and micronutrients– found in beans – are vital for our stamininety success. It's as simple as that.

Are you interested in a decade or more of added healthy lifespan? I am! And I don't have to be a Seventh-day Adventist in Loma Linda, California, or a vigorous Greek islander, or a rural Okinawan to become a centenarian.

Generate your very own lifestyle of good food, Vitamin P with beans (such as in that famous, plant-heavy "Mediterranean Diet"). Add a little red wine, quality olive oil to share with family and friends, plus engage in moderate physical activity. Did I mention that 90-year-old folks and centenarians are growing as a percentage of our general population? Be one of that demographic who youthfully KABOOMs.

Ponce de Leon failed in his quixotic quest to discover the Fountain of Youth. But you and I do not need to fail in our fight against accelerated aging. You and I can concoct our own Fountain of Youth, habitually.

Next, wanna hear about something that is NEAT? I thought so. NEAT is our acronym for "non-exercise activity thermogenesis." In short—our bodies use calories to digest our macronutrients.

NEAT is "energy expended walking to work, typing, performing yard work, undertaking agricultural tasks, and fidgeting. Even trivial physical activities increase metabolic rate substantially"[137] Studies suggest that NEAT may represent about 10 percent of our power produced daily. KABOOMERs are NEAT[138]— trust me.

We neatly:

- Eat more clean macros to avoid obesity (but sadly, *15–25 million baby boomers haven't done this*).
- Eat "relatively" few dairy products and meat macros (like long living Blue Zoners.)
- Eat nuts (if you are free of major allergies and sensitivities) for protein, healthy fats, and fiber. When you enjoy a palmful of nuts, you feel satiated and limit your intake—honest!
- Eat leafy green vegetables. Popeye was right. Take heart with all rainbow-colored fruits and vegetables.
- Enjoy wild, dark-fleshed fish (with high omega-3 levels for your heart health).

Yes, good macro-nutritive items can be found in one's chill box or freezer—like wild salmon or non-farmed shrimp. Good macronutrients don't need to be fresh.

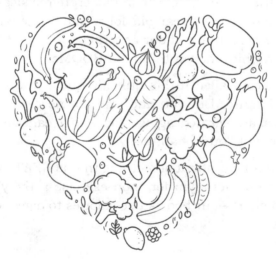

I do my best to exceed our Government's latest dietary guidelines for macro- and micronutrients from Vitamin P because I'm a large, active KABOOMER. I also hedge my bets because our topsoil quantity and quality is not what it used to be. Most of our farmed and grazed topsoil is just plain wimpy for micro-nutrient concentration. So, yes, I take select, supplemental minerals and vitamins. I hope that my chosen brands are what they say they are on labels, incidentally. Even if I don't absorb all my carefully chosen supplements, I'll accept the cost of costlier urine without excess guilt.

Let's address an obvious "macro" point. Digestible protein and essential amino acids are much denser in *meat* than in plants, including so-called superfoods like broccoli. *Quinoa* is an ancient wonder with all nine essential amino acids. Yet, it is "carb heavy" with macro-ratios of carbohydrates to protein. If you find that you want or need to dine on quinoa to meet your intended protein consumption, please note how many grams of carbohydrates come along with that plant source of protein. Speaking of that note:

- Become a savvy food label "scanner." Not obsessive, just savvy. Large food processing companies (yuck) and single source food providers (yeah!) are getting better in their truthful labeling efforts, with help from our big governmental brother. Yet they didn't get large with **Not to Eat** marketing messages.

- Your Koach is *not* a calorie counter. Never has been, and I dunno when I may become one. Very good on you if you are a diligent calorie counter, *if* it helps you on your clean eating journey. Yet I *do* scan food labels for trustworthy nutrition information. Here's why...

Processed Peligro (Danger)

It is sad yet true that many processed foods in our shelved boxes and in (some) frozen food sections are too fatty, too salty and contain too much simple sugar. Did we agree that clean eating is our bullseye to target?

Can eating clean help most of us change our body profile to be more pear-like? True Dat!

We have more, way more, calories stored as fat than we have available as carbohydrates (or muscle) to power our sustained activity. This is important, as some of us are natural "fat burners" or lean ectomorphs, who have metabolic "burn" ratings to stay lean in comparison to their peers. We **need** healthy fats for many bodily functions—yet not too much of 'em!

Many of us are not natural fat burning ectomorphs, and it's not our fault for being mesomorphs or pudgy endomorphs (as illustrated below). A notional ectomorph couple is on the left. Mesomorph friends are centered, and the right-hand couple is endomorphic.

This is a fine pause point to cite the amazing work by Dr. Sylvia Tara regarding fat as a loved and reviled bodily organ. (*The Secret Life of Fat*). My good news/bad news counsel?

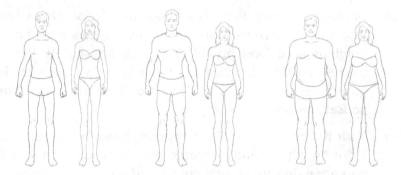

Lean is a four-letter word. Yet it is a good four-letter word. Here's how we should LEAN:

L ighten
  E nhance
    A ctivate
      N urture.

Whatever your natural body type (or somatype), think of being *leaner* as a virtue. Strive to become leaner on your sustained journey with clean eating. Why? Humans' leaner lives tend to be longer ones. And leaner folks tend to be more vital in their activities of daily life. Eat cleaner—and you *can* achieve leaner! I didn't say that this achievement was easy; but I did mention that an added decade on this crazy planet was a viable KABOOMER goal. Yes, this mesomorphic Koach does strive for this. And yes, you can too.

Reiterating another good 4-letter word: *PEAR*. No offense to Georgia *peach*es, but KABOOMER *PEAR*s limit their dangerous and damaging belly fat through clean diets, exercise, de-stressing, *and* restful sleep.

Think of "posifit" *pear* shapes in these four ways to inspire you to fight **dangerous or deadly** fat at your midsection:

P ositive
E mbody
A ttractive
R omantic.

More about *PEAR*s in a bit....Meanwhile, speaking of our exercise fuel and resting results...

Energy and Metabolism
Potential energy from ingested macronutrients is *stored* in our fat cells, our muscles, and our liver. Potential energy is temporarily cached in our amazing bloodstream, to be converted into motion, work—and yes, watts or joules. The fitter we are, the better energy conversions we receive from carbohydrate, fat or protein sources in our heavenly bodies.

Our ingestion and absorption process for endured living is called *metabolism:*[139]

"the process by which your body converts what you eat and drink into energy.

During this complex biochemical process, calories in food and beverages are combined with oxygen to release energy your body needs to function."

Sunlight plus oxygen equates to our thriving and striving functions. Be energized. Let it rip.

We are, quite naturally, what we eat, in both the macro-sense and the micro-sense. That is how we got to now, after millions of years of human development. So, let's think **small** for our second significant class of sustenance.

II. Micronutrients

"Failing to get even those small quantities virtually guarantees disease like heart disease, type 2 diabetes, cancer, and osteoporosis."[141] Don't fail!

We *need* micronutrients. These *small quantities* include minerals and little compounds called vitamins, which we must ingest (or in two special cases which we generate internally) to thrive.

Repeat after your Koach, assuming, that is, that you are interested in living long and well:

a. I will get and absorb **vitamins,** which are *essential* for my normal cell function, growth, and development.

b. I will ingest and absorb **minerals** to keep my bones, muscles, heart, and brain working properly. Minerals are essential for me to *manufacture* needed enzymes and hormones.

Did your Koach mention that micronutrients are *very* important for extended desire and libidinous performance? Guys, as one example, the big O(mega-3) can help you get that pleasurable and healthy other "O" that rhymes with spasm. You will find that micronutrients help men *perform to relax* and *women relax to perform.*

Micronutrients Are Mandatory

You know micronutrients are smaller than macros—yes? I also wager that you realize how critical "micros" are for our quest to live long and well. Think minerals and vitamins—most from plants and soil—Vitamin P. Avoid these at your own peril.

I commend a Center for Disease Control reference for dietary vitals that are small, yet *mighty* (www.cdc.gov/nutrition/micronutrient-malnutrition/micronutrients/index.html): "vital to development, disease prevention, and wellbeing. Micronutrients are not produced in the body and must be derived from the diet. Deficiencies in micronutrients such as iron, iodine, vitamin A, folate, and zinc can have devastating consequences."

KABOOMERs avoid devastation? *Low zinc = low libido.* Granted, one *can* get too much iron or potassium, naturally or via supplementation. Spies kill other spies with potassium injections, after all. Yet it is very difficult to overdose or "OD" on micronutrients—at least for 99.999 percent of us. Your Koach is more concerned about you getting adequate micronutrients.

Health Supplements, Anyone?

I judiciously take vitamin and mineral supplements for my mind and body parts to live my very active life. Just one example is *Magnesium*. I do not take "all-in-one" multivitamins. Rather I take discrete vitamins and minerals. I also eat plenty of Macros with colorful Vitamin P. Yet my muscles crave more than the government-specified minimum daily requirement. After all, I'm not a Gaussian-curved Jill or Jack. I'm a healthy outlier. And you should be one too. I choose my supplement vendor(s) wisely. I buy products that I can trust. That includes supplemental micros (without processing chemicals or contaminants) that should reach my bloodstream and to be absorbed by my cells.

Dietary supplement sales are a huge business in America. Marketers and salesmen know that "we" emulate Don Quixote when it comes to "dreaming the impossible dream." Most dream of presto-change wellness, hoping to see amazing results with supplement-induced fat loss in amazingly short timeframes. Be your own judge and jury about supplementation, please.

And you can, and should, check out published articles asserting that dietary supplementation for micronutrients is overrated. It may be true that vitamins can become "expensive urine," at least for water-soluble vitamins, that is. Folks, I am *no* Nobel laureate when it comes to specifying vitamin dos and don'ts. I am as skeptical as you about supplementation benefits suggested in mice trials, or limited sample size studies with homo sapiens. So, what do I do?

I monitor my personal *pro-neutral-con* reactions to my "mini-trials" of micro-nutrient dosages and frequencies. Then I monitor my quality of life/physical performance for a month or so. Then I may maintain my "micro" nutrient habit or adjust it for better performance. I am confident, from annual laboratory tests of my urine and blood samples, that my measured micros *are* in healthy ranges. If that were not so, I could take proactive steps to address "deficiencies" (per doctor's orders, of course). Thanks, Doc, for those data results! Are both nature and nurture contributors to my reasonable "fortune"? Yup, I am a fortunate son, plus I remember to hedge my wellness "bets" with select smarty pills for minerals and vitamins as my micronutrients. It's not what you ingest; it's what you *absorb!* Did you know that your absorbed magnesium (a very good and necessary micro) may not be well-represented in your drawn blood results? Now, remember the *Wizard of Oz.*

Over the Rainbow

Be a wizardly one. Here's your somehow to get over your Rainbow: Anti-aging diet experts advocate eating *at least five* measured servings of varied fruits and vegetables daily. Does five servings sound like too big of a shopping and eating effort for you? If it does, think again. Prospects for longer and healthier lives are predicated on *muchas frutas y vegetales.*

Start early (time-dependent on your regular breaking of the fast, or whether you are intermittently fasting). Just one example: pop kale or spinach into your breakfast omelet to get started with green *superfoods* and to help you better metabolize the *choline* in your eggs. That wasn't hard, was it? Enjoying avocado on whole grain toast isn't too difficult either. Then stay at it. Munch on organic (if organic produce is affordable for you) colorful carrots, broccoli, and/or plum tomatoes for your snacks. Have fruit and cheese for dessert. You can and should perform **"phyto-magic."** Rainbow food items, when chosen correctly for fiber and glycemic index, *won't* spike your insulin levels. And they can counter big Boomer problems of metabolic syndrome and obesity.

Why this emphasis on color variety for your fruits and vegetables? You might believe a Harvard MD more than me: **"Eat all of the colors of the rainbow,"** [143] says Dr. Michelle Hauser, a clinical fellow at Harvard Medical School. "These colors signal the presence of diverse phytochemicals and phytonutrients.... People who eat diets rich in (plant) phytonutrients have lower rates of heart disease and cancer — the two leading causes of adult death in our United States of America. As a bonus for us, vegetables provide fiber, which helps to prevent constipation and helps to keep cholesterol in check."

Thank you, Dr. Hauser. And thank you, Scientific American writers[144] for piling on"...there is no harm in adding more so-called anti-inflammatory ingredients to your diet."

How does a KABOOMER get his or her anti-inflammatory and immunity boosting Vitamin P?

Mix, juggle, eat them raw, cook them al dente. You can become a phytonutrient pro. Right, phyto means plants. Note: A comprehensive list of colored fruits and vegetables (including white ones omitted from roygbiv hues) can be viewed at www. disabled.com/fitness/nutrition/fruits-veggies/colored.php. It is surely sound advice to eat colorfully!

What Is Sound Nutrition?

Do check this handy dandy summary of sound nutrition at mynutrition.wsu.edu/nutrition-basics/: "As we age, our bodies don't absorb certain vitamins and minerals as well from diet alone. Not to mention, we become more complacent and tend not to cook as often, and therefore eat out more when there aren't any children to feed." [145]

Let's delve into key gap-fillers for stamininety, starting with a baker's dozen of vitamins. Did you know that a Polish researcher named Funk coined the term vita(life)min(amine)? He (wrongly) thought that amino acids were in these tiny life-supporting substances—substances that we need in order to develop and function normally—at any age. How can you get yours?

Ingest and Absorb 13 "Micro" Vitamins However You Can!

Vitamin C and our great group of B vitamins (thiamine, riboflavin, niacin, pantothenic acid, biotin, vitamin B-6, vitamin B-12, and folate) are water-soluble. Why are eight of our essential 13 vitamins in this B group? Scientists like to confuse us. And you might rightly inquire: "What happened to vitamins F, G, H, I, and J in our micro-alphabetical sequence?" That answer is beyond my micro-sustenance expertise. I am not a registered dietitian, nor a nutritional expert. I'm just sharing what I absorb.

Feel free to check Healthline (www.healthline.com/ nutrition/fat-soluble-vitamins) as a robust, reliable source for pluses and minuses of our dietary and metabolic catalysts called vitamins. Or visit Dr. Weil's online resource. Key vitamin and selected mineral hacks are highlighted below. *I list details of all micronutrients on my website (wellpastforty.com).*

I cite 3 "B" vitamins and Vitamin C as "life" amines that do not get stored in our cells, being water soluble. *Remember this as another reason to hydrate!*

BBs

- **B3**: If you have sun-generated skin damage, as I do, Vitamin B3 (Niacinamide) is documented to counter the body's generation of pre-cancer keratoses, and this form does not cause facial flushing. My Dermatologists sold me on the benefits of taking Vitamin B3, as I've had plenty of sun damage and resultant skin cancers.

- **B7**: Biotin is a very critical "B" vitamin for healthy hair and skin. As we age, we don't produce enough collagen to prevent wrinkling and aged skin/hair. Biotin is a key enabler in the production of collagen. Does that resonate? I assert that quality Biotin has been very, very good for me in this century.

- **B12**: Too many adults absorb *too little* B12 as an "animal-based" micronutrient. Vegetarians should monitor their **B12** levels and possibly consider supplementation. It gets more difficult to absorb B12 as we age, Then, many "gut" conditions and prescribed medications make absorption even more difficult. If red blood cell and new DNA production are important to you—absorb adequate B12.

C

- I don't like the thought of scurvy, so I ensure that I get my daily Vitamin C from food and occasional supplements. I don't drink juices, except for tomato juice. I get my Vitamin C from whole citrus fruit (which is easy for a Californian with trees in his yard). And tomatoes. And make a note to ingest zest of lemons or other citrus fruits.

ADEK

- Four *fat soluble* vitamins, Vitamin A (retinol), D, E, and K, are retained at our cellular level. Note: These vitamins need us to ingest healthy macronutrient *fats* for their magic to work! Yes, concentrations of fat-soluble vitamins can build up in our bodies; but would be difficult to ingest/absorb quantities that would cause us problems. Think of Vitamin D, as generated from about 20 minutes per day of sunlight in mid-latitude zones, as an essential example. Vitamin D, particularly in its D3 form, whether from sunlight or supplementation, is key to our muscle metabolism. Am I correct you appreciate muscles?

Our amazing bodies, when properly chugging along, can *manufacture* two fat-soluble vitamins —D (after daylight exposure) and K—yup!

Are there interactions between and among fat-soluble vitamins? Yes, there can be. Vitamin E can adversely affect Vitamin A and K levels if its level is too high. Yet Vitamin E is a great antioxidant to deal with free radicals generated by sunburn, stress, smoking and exercise (you read that correctly—exercise causes free radical "rust" in our bodies). What does Big Government advise us about dosages for these catalysts?

Minimum Daily Requirements (MDRs) or **Recommended Daily Allowances** (RDAs)

Our government and health officials have established MDRs and RDAs for "average Jills and Joes" in our population. That might be fine for many. Yet I'm not average—in either mean, median, or mode analytics. I am bigger, and more active, than statistical means for American male adults. I gladly offer what the results of my healthy trial-and-error for natural supplementation were and are.

Years matter. Absorption changes. Our boomer bodily chemical functions may need tune-ups or natural boosts. My opinion: You know the similarity between an opinion and an @#$hole, yes? Everybody has one.

Folks would need to try very hard to overdose (OD) on micronutrients. It can happen, and acute or chronic doses can harm. I know that I can bump my potassium levels to an upper bound (as measured by blood draw results) if I have enjoyed mangos, oranges and potent mega-vitamins for weeks/months. I'm not too worried about micro–OD, and you don't need to be either.

Does it matter *when* you take vitamins/micronutrients?

You bet. Catalysts must have reactants present for biochemistry to work and to help you stay healthy. Take vitamins with your planned meals if you are in doubt as to whether you are getting your share of these *absorbed* vitamins. Koach, does H_2O matter too? Yes.

III. Water

Our third nutrient class for sustenance is cool, clear, clean water. Every boomer's need for H_2O is different, yet a reasonable body percentage of water weight to total body weight is 45 percent to 55 percent. If you and I don't hydrate, we are very likely to get sick and to under-perform in mind and body, and we may face heat-related conditions.

Drink before thirst! When you note thirst—your fluids dipstick is about a quart low. Yup, and who likes a low dipstick? Yes, water ingested from food items counts. After all, watermelon is almost 90 percent water (and it is an aphrodisiac).

A 135-pound lady boomer should maintain at least 55 pounds of H_2O for her proper bodily function, or her gut won't process food properly. Her skeletal muscles, with 40 percent or more water weight won't perform well if dehydrated.

Aqua vitae! Water is life. Do *not* stay thirsty, my friends.

Drumroll...drink at least eight glasses (cups) of "pure" water daily (eight x eight oz. in shorthand). Sip throughout the day until your urine is quite light. (Vitamins and some foods like red beets may occasionally cause a darker hue in your urine.) No worry there. Just strive for 8x8 glasses of water or more daily in order to thrive! Salud!

You are "mostly" water by weight. Mostly, as in about 50 percent or more as a percentage of overall body weight. Taking sustenance to the limit, we know that men or women will die from dehydration long before they will perish from starvation. Proper hydration is a must for everyone, yet more so for us who exercise and stay active. Remember Dr. Meerman's TED counsel: active folks exhale lots of water vapor. Fill 'er up.

Listen to my cheers…humans now drink more bottled water than soda pop! 'Bout time!

Water is wonderful as a solvent. By this I mean that water-soluble vitamins couldn't serve as our performance catalysts if we didn't have bodily water to help them metabolize.

Water is also essential as our air conditioning system. Water can absorb a whole bunch of exercise-generated heat so that we can still function when weather get a little sticky.

Mollifying hangovers or less obvious reasons for drinking at least 64 ounces of water throughout your days are offered by Greatist.com[147] and highlighted here:

12 KABOOMER Reasons to Drink

1. Balance bodily fluids
2. Caloric control
3. Muscle fuel (Dehydration is a *key* factor in degraded performance.)
4. Clearer skin
5. Kidney function (Our pair of kidney filters work on over 200 quarts of blood daily! Water helps flush the waste that every Boomer generates.)
6. Boost productivity

7. Fight fatigue
8. Hangover helper
9. Pain prevention
10. Regulate bowel movements
11. Fight illness
12. Boost clear thinking.

"Keep a water bottle handy at all times."

Make that a non-BPA, plastic-free bottle, if you please.

Water makes us *who we are*—hydrated vibrant KABOOM-ERs, who can exercise with less fatigue and stay cool by drinking "before thirst." If I waited until I sensed thirst to hydrate, I couldn't perform at my best. You may already be a quart low on vital water when you sense thirst. At least when exercising, *sip ahead of your thirst!* That is because partial dehydration is a prominent reason for fatigue and under-performing. That "sipping ahead of thirst" is also important because our amazing bodies can *only* absorb one liter (about a quart) of water per hour.

For average-size adults engaged in moderate athletic activity, there isn't much of a need to imbibe water during your session if your workout is for an hour or less in duration. Can you spell *hyponatremia*? It is rare, yet possible, to drink *too much* water if an essential electrolyte—sodium—in our blood and body becomes too diluted.

This condition can kill—honest—by exercise-associated hyponatremia (abbreviated as EAH). And for another heated hydration topic, Safety....

Call 911

Please learn to recognize possible symptoms of two heat-related illnesses: heat exhaustion and heat stroke.[148] When in doubt, call 911 and seek immediate medical help!

1. Early warning signs of **heat exhaustion** are nausea,

light-headedness, fatigue, muscle cramping and dizzi-
ness.

Conversely...

2. Someone experiencing **heat stroke** may have a head-
ache, confusion, no sweating, rapid heart rate, nausea or vomiting, and may lose consciousness. If a heat
stroke is suspected, it is vital to act:

- Call 911 immediately
- Move the person to a cooler place
- Use cold compresses to get body temperature down
- Do **not** give fluids!

If you become a bystander and possibly a first responder
to someone with a heat-related illness, please know when offering water to the sufferer is a **no-no!** Water for heat stroke
sufferers is verboten. Counterintuitive, yet possibly fatal! See
www.webmd.com/first-aid/understanding-heat-related-ill-
ness-symptoms for details.

Shifting supplemental gears... Tell me, Koach, can I skip
supplements for *micronutrients*?

Perhaps. Get as much of your macro- and micronutrients
from wholesome natural diets as possible. Yet, I hedge my
vitality bet! I do not hesitate to ingest *clean* supplemental vitamins and minerals if my lab specimens suggest that I'm not
absorbing enough. I also do not hesitate to selectively ingest
more micros than an average Jack or Jill in our demographic.
I don't consider myself as *average*. That's affordable and prudent term insurance in my physical chart of accounts!

Make a note. It may take weeks to bump "low" levels of micronutrients to healthy levels. Good *non-trivial* things do take
time.

Trivial Pursuit? Not! Sleep, anti-stress efforts, *and clean
sustenance* comprise *two-thirds* of our successful campaign
to gain stamininety. I think of those critical success factors

as enablers for me to move and sweat, whatever the breakout percentage is for our success recipe to thrive and strive. In KABOOMER circles of life, habitual exercise helps us sleep better; it counteracts some of the stresses of modern life; and it nudges us to eat *healthier* because chemical messengers like anti-fat leptin, testosterone, and our natural growth hormones ramp up after we sweat.

A similar circle of life exists for sustenance. Macronutrients, micros, and water sustain our muscle fibers so that we can *KABOOM*. Our clean eating enables our restful Z's. Proper food fuels our bedrock endurance efforts. And right foodstuffs help us achieve high percentages of vital body tissue while lowering body percentages of pernicious white fat.

These interrelated and supportive enablers for stamininety are best achieved with attitude, perseverance and a bit of scientific knowledge. Chances are darned slim that you'll party past 90 if you have dietary habits like James Galdofini, or the Mick:

> "If I'd known I'd live this long, I'd have taken better care of myself."—Mickey Mantle, a damned NY Yankee

Our sustenance habits are not trivial pursuits. We eat well to live long and well (with a little bit of luck, that is). Help your liver work well and keep your gastro-intestinal tract (a.k.a. "gut") thriving. Keep both pears and apples in your non-trivial gunsights. Here is your what, why, how and WIFM station for these fruit shapes: "Apple" belly fat is unhealthy. "Apple" excess belly fat inflames our 4F systems. What experts call "central obesity" is akin to a life-threatening cancer for those whose measured waists are larger than hips.

As a shapely reality, I implore you to pursue a pear-shaped body. Pear-shaped? Yes, strive for this silhouette or shape, rather than a rounded apple-shaped body. Pear-shaped, meaning that your visceral fat and central obesity is low enough that your hip circumference is notably bigger than your waist. *This is a key.* Lower your belly fat as best as your stamininety habits, unique endocrine system and genetic makeup allow. Two "figures" below suggest those two fruity shapes as wake-up calls with life and death implications for all. We'll shortly revisit a scary relationship: **central obesity and white fat are linked to cellular aging, inflammation and *cancer*.**

Apple and Pear Shapes

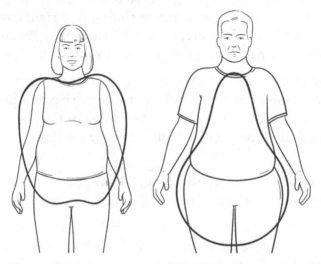

These two notional boomers are likely Endomorphs, with apparent bodily fat in excess. Yet, the apple-shaped woman may be at greater risk for chronic metabolic syndromes and early deaths than the male "pear-shaped" guy to her left in the Figure. Location, location, location....

Fruit shape and central obesity are key for boomers from both planets: Mars and Venus. Yes, the **smaller** your waist-to-hip ratio, the better you appear, and the better you perform by day and night. KABOOM. If you have too big a waist (as an *apple*), some of the longevity and vitality odds are stacked *against* you. As for too big a waist in relation to your hip circumference, then you may have metabolic syndrome effects, with nasty outcomes. The Mayo Clinic offers these outcomes from *woeful* weight at your waist:[149] "heart disease, stroke and type 2 diabetes, increased blood pressure, high blood sugar, and abnormal (high) cholesterol or triglyceride levels." Wowza.

What icons of our youthful days had impressive waist-to-hip ratios and "hourglass" or pear silhouettes? Yup. Barbie and Ken. **Know** the ***do or die*** measure of your waist-to-hip ratio. This table shows statistical ranges of pear-ness that you can consider as your *do or die* goals:

Waist-to-Hip Ratios and Risk

Health risk	Women	Men
Low	0.80 or lower	0.95 or lower
Moderate	0.81–0.85	0.96–1.0
High	0.86 or higher	1.0 or higher

Source: www.healthline.com/health/waist-to-hip-ratio and a calculator at www.healthstatus.com/calculate/waist-to-hip-ratio

Key Notes:

1. Waist to Height Ratios (WtHR) are also associated with health risk. You can use Dr. Google or call your KA-BOOMER Koach if you'd like to check your Waist to Height Ratios.

2. Blow off BMI! I mean that. Body mass indicators are misleading for many healthy, lean, and muscular KA-BOOMERs. Trust me. To heck with you, Dr. Quetelet, and to hell with your flawed 1830s statistics for today's body mass. Make a note: Work your waist to hip ratios and blow off BMI. Period. Now, let's raise a glass and toast geroprotectors.

Clean eating and sipping may indeed serve as our "geroprotection" to age slower. A very good thing, right? Noble grapes in wine can help put phytonutrient "time in a bottle" (thank you, Jim Croce). Wine's plant-based nutrients have fancy names like resveratrol and polyphenols. Simply put—wine can help our mood, heart health and mind—if we heed Satchel Paige's and Grandma's caution about moderation. Moderate drinking can be a sustaining habit to help you gain stamininety, whether you can spell resveratrol or polyphenol or not.

Granted: smoking, chronic diseases like diabetes, and solitude may have higher actuarial impact on your longevity than clean eating. Yet unhealthy dietary habits that we can and should control are certain life takeaways. *Are extra years of what you can control important to you?*

Sure, you face temptations, though in different garden ways than Adam and Eve faced. **Avoid** these seven edible temptations, and *don't* accept offers from serpents:

1. Anything artificial (e.g., food coloring)
2. High fructose corn Syrup (HFCS)
3. Household toxins
4. Preservatives
5. Trans fats
6. Alcohol in excess
7. Mono-sodium glutamate (MSG).

Avoid 'em if you want to stay in a safe passing lane. Else, highway danger!

Highway to Your Danger Zone

Thanks, Kenny Loggins, for your amped-up anthem.

- Don't burn red meat to charred well-done intensity. If you char it, skip it or feed it to Fido.

- Don't forget your far-from-the-edge Vitamin P to aid our body's largest gland, the liver.

- Don't burn your liver: As the largest gland in your amazing body, a liver keeps us from toxic danger zones—if we don't keep it on afterburn like Maverick did in *Top Gun*. We are blessed that our livers are extraordinary filters for many environmental and dietary bad boys. Kudos to our department of sanitation!

The fact that livers do many other useful things—like store glycogen and process fats to support our motion and muscle— is amazing! So why make it harder for our livers to naturally detoxify our bodies? Hmmm...can our lives extend longer and be better with "sanitation" and lower pollutant-triggered estrogen levels? KABOOM. To counter liver burnout, eat plenty of Vitamin P products, like avocados, and seeds that are high in oleic acid. Did you know that coffee can mitigate our liver's inflammation?

Next, lets acknowledge known and unknown impacts of plastics on fish and mammal livelihood (including us).

One Word: Plastics

Don't fall for the love story of Americans and plastics (read more in Susan Freinkel's excellent book *Plastic: A Toxic Love Story*). Contrary to counsel for Ben Braddock in *The Graduate*, plastics are not good for our marine life, or for us. Plus, most of us suspect that plastics are unhealthy for us as when used in food and drink *packaging* and *microwaving*. We thankfully live in a world that is less reliant on plastics and *more* conscious of environmental damages than in the last century, at least in developed nations like ours. Yet, consumer and clean eater beware!

The half-life of microplastic beads in our oceans can range up to hundreds of years![150] Did your catch of ocean shrimp taste a bit bumpy? I hope not!

Guys, are you concerned that our environmental pollutants and plastics can raise your estrogen levels? You should be!

This KABOOMER eats foods that experts say counter pollutants (naturally). Here is vital Vitamin P (again):

"Eating *more than two cups* of broccoli, cabbage, cauliflower, kale, or other cruciferous veggies a day is associated with a *20-percent reduced risk of dying*, compared to eating one-third of a cup a day, or less. The cruciferous compound *sulforaphane* is a powerful inducer of our **detox** enzymes."[151]

You Don't Say

Do *not* neglect what our National Institute of Health states about eating to live long and well:[152]

"Vegetables, fruits, and soy products are rich in antioxidants that are essential to lower disease risk stemming from reactive oxygen systems in the body. Green and black teas are excellent sources of antioxidants of a polyphenol nature, as are cocoa and some chocolates. *Nutritional lifestyles that offer the possibility of a healthy long life can be adopted by most populations in the world.*"

Sound simple for us at our Medicare ages? Yet over and over in life, I've learned that simple things are truly hard to sustain. Here is another tip: Don't forget about food sensitivities and allergies!

Ahchoo!

I am also blessed that any of my (known) food allergies are minor. No EpiPen carried (yet). I have several low-grade allergies, which include throat scratches and sneezes from some nuts (cashews) and some spices. This acknowledged awareness is what it is, because spices are *good* for most of us. I prudently keep at it, using spice because I should. Cinnamon is a fine surrogate for simple sugar, as an example.

I suppose that I could survive an iodine sensitivity for shellfish, yet my life without shrimp and grits would be uncomfortably different for me. I will bet several nickels (which is quite a wager for this cheapskate Vermonter) that we gain more food sensitivities, or see 'em manifested, as we get older (*not old*). Just keep paddling up your variety creek. Find clean and healthy food choices that don't make you sneeze or cough on your healthful journey. One example is that our peers with asthmatic symptoms should choose "no sulfite-added" wines to avoid breathing problems.

Eat Clean = Live a longer, fuller, happier, better, more productive, more meaningful Life!

This plainly means: more time with your partner, kids, grandkids, loved ones, friends; more time for the things you love to do, the projects you want to finish, the places you want to see...Ways to live your best life the way you were intended to live it for as long as you are intended to live it.

***Do not forget* that diet is likely a leading cause of death in America!**

Take your self-assessed look at *unforgettable* diet factors and death:

1. Try the *Living To 100 Life Expectancy Calculator* which also factors in your zip code for air quality, sun exposure, traffic and lifestyle demographics: *www.living-to100.com/*

2. Or work a TIME magazine estimator: time.com/3485579/when-will-i-die-life-expectancy-calculator/

I don't know when I will die, but being the last partier standing appeals to me!

Move, engage in resistance activity, chill out, sweat, and sleep. Eat clean because our mind, body, and gut *know* what is good for performance and survivability. Sure, many, as in millions, have glandular or hormonal imbalances. Yet almost everyone can do better! Almost everyone, at least those *without* early death wishes, should lower visceral fat and increase activity!

A reminder: Four special Elephants that can squash your "clean eating" are addressed in Addenda after your Kool Down Chapter:

1. Metabolic Syndrome
2. Gut (a.k.a. microbiome): whether healthy or leaky
3. Unhealthy Fat
4. Diets.

Don't get squashed. Let's take a cleansing breath as we call it a clean sweep.

CHAPTER 9

Kool Down

"If you would not be forgotten, as soon as you are dead and rotten, either write things worth reading, or do things worth writing."—*Poor Richard's Almanack*

Mindful of that bon vivant, Ben Franklin, I tried to write *things worth reading* for you. **KABOOMER: Thriving and Striving into your 90s** was certainly worth writing! My own phoenix years and encounters since 2001 certainly offered me "things worth writing" about. Certainly, you are my judge and jury for whether (or not) I'll be forgotten.

Kudos! You made it through all seven munificent steps to help you gain stamininety. To form memorable habits for thriving and striving. You learned about my research and experiential lessons that increase your odds for living long and living well.

You now hold practical ways to walk the KABOOMER walk (and take steps two at a time), with or without my further Koaching.

Now, kool down, stretch, and hydrate a bit. Treat your body as a temple or as a special shrine. Give yourself a well-deserved shoulder hug and a good morning stretch to lengthen your posterior chain. Please drink some low-fat or full-fat (four percent) chocolate milk post-workout as part of your good eating habits. And consider a *nappucino* or *nooner* to nip stress and fatigue. Laugh often. Move to sweat and push/pull stuff as good medicine.

A revered TV and radio personality, Charles Osgood, has retired to a French villa. He assuredly enjoys a Mediterranean lifestyle and vintage, noble grapes. Thinking about messieurs Franklin and Osgood; each has enjoyed a good life and has helped others' build vital and vibrant lives. Perhaps I can be so lucky, *although I haven't spent much time in France.* But I do spend time helping others live longer and better, as my pleasure. Back to our expat, Charles Osgood. Among his many accomplishments is a written **Responsibility Poem** [153] (www.greatexpectations.org/Websites/greatexpectations/images/pdf/lp/responsibility/Responsibility%20poems.pdf.

This, in my humble opinion, fits your (and my) journeyed road and daily habits. I quote, in part:

> "There was a most important job that needed to be done, and no reason not to do it, there was absolutely none.
> But in vital matters such as this, the thing you ask is this: who exactly will it be who'll carry out the task?
> Anybody could have told you that Everybody knew that *this was something **Somebody would surely have to do.**"*

*Anybody, everybody, **somebody** and/or nobody*—hmm. I strive to walk the talk of being a *somebody*. As a KABOOMER who takes his wellness job seriously, yet not too seriously. I truly hope that you might also be that *somebody* to get an *important* job like stamininety done. You surely should; if your goal is to put life in your years and add years to your life. A longer and better life as an encore performance for your loved ones and for you.

Half of KABOOMER was written in the longish church season of Epiphany. So, I am grateful to listen and learn from a marvelous orator who doubles as our parish rector. Once her words, which often serve as an epiphany or eureka moment for me, included a familiar New Testament passage. I bet that millions of us know this one: "Love is patient, love is kind...". Not bad counsel for a parable that is twenty centuries old! Change, commitment, plus spending time on what really matters are the priest's timely themes that I wish to share. Later in this Corinthians chapter, there is a phrase about "giving up childish ways."

Don't give up the playful and fun ways of little ones. Why shouldn't we be *young at heart and body?* Can you give up your old ways, and start refreshed with your new wellness routines and healthy habits? Can you commit to play, and work to put years in your life plus life in your years?

The Answers Are Yes!

Let's each strive to be that **somebody** who parties past 90. James Salter wrote, "life passes into pages if it passes into anything."[154] Make your passages vibrant, since we KABOOMERs do **not** let life pass into plain 'ol pages.

Surely, striving for stamininety can be challenging. Particularly if you start from a reasonably low level and want to move to incremental or competitive levels of strength fitness. And when aches, pains, bumps, and bruises are passengers on our travels. Remember Ben Franklin and Nietzsche when your motivation slips a bit. Never forget the power of a smile or a chuckle.

Chuckle along with Judith Viorst whom chronicles both joys and humor of aging well. Judith isn't one of us by chronological age, yet she shares our KABOOMER spirit! One of her humorous books is entitled **Nearing 90**. We *should* aspire to thrive near 90 and beyond. Thereafter, your KABOOMER's extraordinary epitaph will summarize your life well-lived.

Yes, thus ends my homily. As I head off to my tub to soak in Epsom salts and wind down for restorative sleep, I sign off with this "last right:"

> "Whether you think you can or think you cannot—you are right." —*Henry Ford*

Thank you and **be right**. KABOOM.

/s/

Dave Frost
KABOOMER Koach

Addenda

Addendum A

Stairway to Stamininety

Let's agree to agree that it is best to begin with your goals and aspirations as Covey's "end in mind." Surely these "stretch" goals can and should be updated as your "party past 90" journey progresses. Let's also agree that nearly every one of us 75 million baby boomers in the good ol' U.S. of A. has: a chink in our armor, a joint that isn't quite what it once was, a little less gumption to keep on keepin' on, or some other reality of modern maturity. But we don't despair!

We, in this 75-million demographic of Woodstock's "flower children" are alive and kicking, stepping or striding. Hopefully sleeping restfully and de-stressing with laughter often. And eating clean.

We have great things to accomplish before we're put in an urn or deposited six feet underground. (I ask that my remains be scattered at sea when my days are done.) We are truly blessed to have "modern medicine" on our side. We generate our own blessings with healthy sustaining habits to fend off the Grim Reaper's appearance—Lady Luck and your own creator willing, of course.

The following table is your "do" list to refresh, restore, and grow in that amazing corpus of yours—with its extraordinarily evolved biochemistry and kinetics as blessings. Please think of these table entries as "hacks"—rather than as platitudes or bromides.

Always remember that little green guy in Star Wars' early segments. The Jedi Yoda offered: "Do or Do Not. There is no Try."

I won't add a Try column in this Dos and Don'ts checklist because of him. I won't add a Neutral column either. KABOOMER wellness is about driving forward (in some kinetic and biochemical gear)—and not slipping into reverse or idling in neutral. Please think about that—and perhaps even adapt this analogy as a mantra or affirmation—whether you drive a Tesla or a Ford F-150: "I won't get stuck in neutral or slip into reverse!"

DOs and DON'Ts on your Stairway to Stamininety

	DOs	DON'Ts
1. Sleep	a. Find your way to ensure approximately 7 hours of restful and restorative sleep daily. b. Keep your bedroom or sleeping quarters cool (64–68 degrees F.). c. Verify if you have a sleep disorder or condition (apnea?)—like 20+ million boomers do. Right—about one out of every three of us! CPAPs save lives. 1. Try a cool shower or warm soak 75-90 minutes before lights out. e. Stretch just a bit. 1. Find your "ideal" sleep position, adding pillows or props as prudent. g. Generate melatonin naturally, or episodically use a tiny melatonin pill to get you into deep sleep.	a. Prolong screen time before pillow time (TV, tablet, smart phone). b. Concede to "I can't sleep" patterns. You have at least "some" sleep matters which you can control. c. Neglect a professional audit for your mattress, bed mite cover, pillow. These items matter, trust me. d. Skip free resources—like sleep.org. e. Smoke in bed—after your romp. f. Forget that sleep time is restoration AND calorie-burn time!

	DOs	DON'Ts
2. Stability	a. Master your own Question of Balance. b. Learn about a big word with big implications: Proprioception. Sure, a sobriety check by the law is also proprioception. Yet knowing where your body parts are spatially is important now and later. c. Try that longevity test often: single leg stands with eyes closed (15 seconds for each leg). d. Advance to asymmetric/ unbalanced moves and activities when ready. e. Spend time in your bare feet and work your big (great) toes.	a. Fall! Duh.... b. Avoid "right" exercise and activity regimens because of conditions (e.g., COPD, multiple sclerosis (MS), type 2 diabetes). c. c. Lose your "on guard" vigilance for tripping, slipping, body-torqueing hazards. d. Wear "pillows" on your feet all the time. e. Forget that stability is your everyday imperative.

	DOs	DON'Ts
3. Stamina	a. Get to your glisten or sweat stages from activity or workouts. You need the "right" intensity and longevity to stimulate your cytokine messengers for wellness and longevity. b. Seek the "runner's high" for natural endorphin production. c. Mix it up! Don't just stick with your same ol' "dreadmill" or same swimming pool laps. Seek fresh air and new sights for your mindful motion. d. Invest most of your endurance days at low intensity. Even when you are ready, one weekly Tabata or other High Intensity Interval Training (HITT) session is adequate. Trust me. e. Celebrate your slow-twitch fiber. You can hang in there with young whippersnappers for endurance more than in "plyometrics" or in fast-twitch fiber activities.	a. "Fly then Die" in a single workout or activity. Don't neglect your finish line goal. If you miss the mark, try again. b. Spend "too much" time and effort in your twilight zone for training heart rate. c. Expect to optimally gain muscle while gaining endurance in your same periodization. You can achieve both, just not optimally. What are your present goals? d. Forget to check your urine hue and amount produced. If you become dehydrated, you cannot perform at your best AND you may get into a bad "heat" condition! e. Neglect to elevate your heart rate for a total of three hours a week!

	DOs	DON'Ts
4. Strength (Resistance)	a. Resistance-train your whole body (and three planes) twice each week.	a. Concede to sarcopenia (loss of skeletal muscle with age).
	b. See a doctor before you engage in moderate or strenuous resistance training. Get your "PAR-Q" clearance to thicken your sarcomeres.	b. Ladies- don't ignore your need to challenge your skeleton to keep bone density as high as possible (may need calcium supplementation). Swimming is great—yet it doesn't help your bone density—right?
	c. Remember what builds muscle content (essential amino acids for sustenance and repairing muscular fiber micro-tears).	
	d. Acknowledge that resistance is not futile! This is true for nearly all of us boomers. We can and should use bands, phone books, isometrics, travel suitcases—and "metal" to resist when we are ready.	c. Be or become lazy or sedentary. Work is good for humans, and moving heavy things is too.
		d. Forget functional training, like farmer's walks.
	e. Challenge your skeletal muscles, connective tissue, and joints until you are in your senescent 90s.	e. Overlook a training buddy. As boomer band Three Dog Night reminded us, "One is the loneliest number...."
	f. Spend more time and effort on free weights and whole-body efforts, than machine lifts and muscle isolation moves.	f. Try to be animal-strong like an ant, a flea, or grasshopper. Rather do your best as a homo sapiens because your strength matters!

	DOs	DON'Ts
5. Stress - NOT	a. Remember that 95 percent of life is small stuff—so don't sweat those small stuffs. Let it go, let it go! b. Leverage your soft skills—emotional intelligence—to self-realize and self-actualize. You are in control of many things in your life, even if you don't realize it now. c. Monitor your resting heart rate and respiration patterns. You can learn to decompress a situation—all by your lonesome. d. Affirm life with gratitude—regularly. Life is what it is—but life can be good or better if you are grateful. e. Breathe, baby, breathe. f. Try Walden Pond strolls or go for a nature walk. g. Know that some sounds (not jackhammers or jetliners) can mellow you, and/or they can increase your mindfulness. Which tones or "white" noises work for you? h. Get that annual flu vaccine plus all the hepatitis shots you need to remain healthy among bad microbes. i. Remember that it takes you more muscles to frown or scowl than to smile. Your friends like to see your pearly whites, yes? Note to self: Take care of those important dental bones for wellness.	a. Emotionally eat (or drink). b. Stay in your fast lane continually. Boomers are no longer "Energizer bunnies" on nuclear power. c. Pass up golden opportunities to DO NOTHING. It's okay to chill. d. "Live" on social media or get absorbed in unlimited screen time. These are anti-social and anti-wellness avoidances. e. Go through life alone as a hermit. Enjoy tribal connections. f. Forget to turn the other biblical cheek. g. Be a grouch. Sesame Street has one of those characters. We need more jokesters and storytellers to make your and my world better places.

	DOs	DON'Ts
6. Stretching	a. Make mind-body connections—even if you call your stretched position a cat, dirty dog, or cobra instead of a Sanskrit asana. Namaste. b. If you are interested in adventurous romps, review what Kama Sutra poses you can hold and cherish. c. *Strengthen to Lengthen*—daily! d. Invest in a few affordable stretch aids. e. Give yourself a good hug daily. f. Work toward limber capacity—whether that is a slow, deliberate toe touch (with your knees locked), or doing a demanding pistol squat or Turkish get-up with good form. g. Say after me: Sitting is our new smoking hazard. I can find a standing desk or workstation!	a. Ignore your posterior chain (calves, hamstrings, glutes, and lower back (LPHC)). b. Forget that your ball (stability), wall, and floor are your "stretchy" friends. Don't be strangers to them. c. Don't forget to investigate ancient techniques like Qigong, tai Chi, and yoga. Namaste! d. Don't let your stretching routines come up short. Overcome your restrictions in movement from stiff, immobile joints or connective tissues. Don't go it alone: You can access body therapy tools, muscular chain releases for your anterior, posterior, and lateral chains. e. Forget to investigate your affordable options for self-massage and nose-to-toes focus. f. Ask for vigorous massages before your haj, big event, or competitions.

	DOs	DON'Ts
7. Eating Clean	a. Eat to live well. Stick to an 80/20 ratio of good, clean sustenance (five-six days a week). b. Get familiar and then walk your talk of a clean anti-inflammatory lifestyle/diet. This could be your matter of life or untimely death. c. Go "au naturel" if clean, good quality foodstuffs and drinks are both available and affordable for you. d. Try varied eating patterns to fit your lifestyle and goals. e. Remember that the optimal route to great abs is through your pantry and refrigerator door. f. Know that simple sugars and HFCS (high fructose corn syrup) foods are devilish, with known and unknown effects on your wellness. Avoid evil macronutrients!	a. Count calories (unless this process works for you). b. Live a monastic life (unless you are a monk). c. Eat processed foods. d. Skip healthy, plant-based or fishy fats. e. Ignore why Blue Zone centenarians get to their 100 mark. (Being social and eating beans are two reasons—honest). f. Forget what Popeye and Olive Oyl knew.

	DOs	DON'Ts
7. Eating Clean (cont'd.)	g. Take a complimentary vitamin survey to get your individualized scoop on what micronutrient vitamins and minerals might enable your wellness journey. h. Invest in whatever it takes to prudently rev up your metabolism. It may not be your fault that your endocrine system is neutral or negative as you're trying to get along on your journey. Hypo-thyroid linkage to central obesity is one example that you can hopefully counter. i. Eat to be a pear (shaped) body type. j. Learn what type of fat burner you currently are. This makes a difference! k. Ingest adequate fiber (a carb macronutrient) to "move" daily. l. Honor that 50 percent of your bodily temple that is good ol' H2O. Drink cool, clear water throughout your boomer days. **KABOOM !**	g. Forego REGULAR laboratory tests for blood sugar, testosterone (if interested), micronutrients, etc. Muy Importante! It's more what gets absorbed more than what you eat (or what you supplement). h. Let your waist to hip/waist to height measures change for the worse. Apple-shaped boomers (both sexes) are more prone to chronic problems and metabolic syndrome. i. Think that James Galdofini is a right role model for proper diet and lifestyle.

Which path for Do's and Don'ts will you choose? There is time to change the road you're on!

Note: Unless you read a specific callout, these hacks (above) are intended for both female and male Boomers. When I find a collaborative female partner, a published sequel to KABOOM-ER will drill down into what you ladies specifically face in your bespoke journeys for stamininety.

Stay tuned!

Addendum B: Safety

Lift! But Be Careful Out There!

Deb, Garrett, George, and y'all, heed these elements of safe KABOOMER strength and stamina efforts.

Be prudent and safe for your strength and resistance activities.

1. Get your formal MD approval before engaging in strength routines. Better safe than sorry is another platitude that you've heard again and again. You may have seen or may have completed a Physical Aptitude Readiness-Questionnaire (PAR-Q) (eparmedx.com/wp-content/uploads/2013/03/FINAL-FILLABLE-ParQ-Plus-Jan-2019.pdf) before you worked with a fitness trainer like me. This health and wellness checklist is mandatory for older athletes.

2. Know your body and its current capacities to lift, move, and carry objects, or moving to sweat for longish periods.

   a. Get key measurements and know your body type. What is important is to start, and then to extend and expand what you can and will do! Moderation, Satchel Paige offered, is our pacing advice. Don't chase an impossible dream.

   b. Don't pass through a door of discomfort to get an extra repetition or move extra tonnage. Discomfort and pain are feedback to which you must listen.

   c. As one listed strength benchmark, untrained boomers should be able to deadweight lift three-quarters of their body weight one time (1RM). KABOOMERs should do better—safely.

3. Acknowledge that bodily soreness is swell... well, sorta.

   Soreness can be a useful sign of your exerted muscles'

micro-tears, recovery and repair cycle. You need these feedback signals! Soreness is a continual acquaintance of ours, so accept its presence (ensuring that the sensation is not acute or chronic pain, that is). These after-symptoms are requisites for your growth toward stamininety.

4. Accept a bit of the "pain and gain" adage. Not too much, as my key point is do not overdo it. Guys, you won't become an overnight strength success story. Ladies, becoming Ms. Hercules in a fortnight just isn't in those cards you were dealt. Exercise-induced pain signals are telling us something valuable.

Your health professionals should be consulted if any pain becomes acute or chronic for you. Living with pain isn't tickety-boo. Yes, there is a price you'll eventually pay for minor injuries to muscles and joints with work. Yet that cost is better than the close-out price of sarcopenia you will pay if you don't do resistance work.

Protect
Rest
Ice
Compress
Elevate
(Credit: NFPT)

Notes:

1. If something in your musculature or skeleton ails you a wee bit, use something else to keep getting your strength medicine! If you have a wee glitch, do not abstain from resistance training at your own risk. Let's say, as an example, that your left forearm has minor repetitive stress injuries. No worry: for now, you can work the right side unilaterally.

2. If your medical coverage allows—push for physical

therapy—don't do the "guy thing," pressing past and ignoring what pain means or hoping that it will go away.

Acute and chronic injuries are horses of different colors than wee ailments. It is frustrating if a spinal disk is herniated or worse. It is frustrating when your radial nerve flares up and you have *tennis elbow* syndrome as a result. Or when sutured sites are healing after surgery.

I speak firsthand about being out of action for too long due to my herniated disk and "rower's elbow." And shin splints. And plantar fasciitis. Life happens.

Special physical conditions? Ponder multiple sclerosis (MS) or perhaps a foot amputation caused by diabetes. It is usually recommended that you engage in a structured fitness program involving strength/resistance work. That also rings true for prevalent boomer conditions of arthritis. True dat for other adult complications too.... Research. Recruit someone to help you get started; then away you go to get your medicine! GO safely—with these seven practical reminders.

Seven-Up for Safety

Smart folks who work in Harvard Yard advise us[155] to "keep your strength training safe and effective." That is wise counsel. Seven practical reminders to make your strength work **safe** are:

1. Warm up and cool down for five to 10 minutes with dynamic stretching (see our Stretch chapter).
2. Focus on proper form, not weight. Where is your spotter for certain lifts like bench presses?
3. Work at your right tempo to stay in control always.
4. Pay attention to your breathing.
5. Slowly increase weight or resistance for your progressive efforts.
6. Stick with your planned routine.
7. Give your muscles a break with time off for their repair, recovery and growth.

Physio-pedia.com is my trusted reference source[156] when I discuss pain and its management with my clients (and talk to myself).

"Pain is *always subjective*, and each individual learns the application of the word through experiences related to injury in early life.... For people suffering from pain, their initial response is to avoid activity and seek rest. And yet exercise therapy is often prescribed as a treatment option to manage pain."

I ask you to try and manage your pain symptoms with modified exercise rather than *avoiding activity*. Trusty Physio-pedia doesn't mention an elephant in your safety and pain management room; but I will—and that elephant is steroidal supplements for unnatural muscle gain, and coincidentally, with serious prospects for serious side effects.

Again, you do not need fancy, expensive equipment or paraphernalia to push, pull or lift heavy stuff. Tuck that away, for times when travelling, or when gyms are unavailable. Don't spend more dinero than you need for strength training stuff for weightlifting.

So, exercise your rights and be sporty with these three types of lifting activity: 1. Heavy 2. Long 3. Fast. What you perform in each type of (up)lifting activity is good medicine.

And repeat these relational phrases after your Koach:

You can't out-train bad nutrition.

Where the mind goes, the body follows.

Eat well and optimize your mind-body connection, all day every day.

What follows in the next Addendum is your When? Where? and How? details for KABOOMER Resistance Training.

Addendum C

When? Where? and How?

These strength matters answer all 3 queries.

When?

Timing your strength/resistance exercise is dependent on your biorhythm and your intended goal or end games. I commend to you Dan Pink's "Ultimate Guide" for when to exercise, in his eponymously titled book, When.[157]

Drumroll: When should you (generally) pursue strength training, or heavy yard work, or romantic romps? Do you recall that great romping counsel of Jack Nicholson in Bucket List? Some episodic things are not to be wasted.

You might consider mornings as your best work-and-play windows if your fitness goals are to:

1. Lose weight
2. Boost your mood
3. Keep to your routine, or most poignantly for this segment
4. Build strength.

Why? Both ladies' and gentlemen's higher testosterone levels are the prime chemical reason for morning strength sessions. Flag: Please read your concluding testosterone and ADAM addendum for details about this key endocrinal messenger. Testosterone or "T" is an organic chemical messenger ($C_{19}H_{28}O_2$) with just carbon, hydrogen, and oxygen. Nothing too sexy about those elements?! This controller is generated by male testes or by female ovaries, plus adrenal glands for all. Unless an abnormal factor arises, all of us should produce "T" until we stop breathing, though in diminished levels as we age. Testosterone is hopefully, and naturally, present in right concentrations for both men and women who wish to maintain and build skeletal muscle, and to support red blood cell production. **And** to churn butter better, bandicoot, belly-bump (for one position), or better dance in the sheets.

Remember Mr. T on television's A Team? Well, the real Mr. T as a KABOOMER suggests that we "Pity the Fool" who doesn't work naturally to boost his or her T. This alphabet letter T is key to the livelihood of both genders. Yup.

My strong timing? I've found, over my many years, that if I get a workout or pleasant activity done in the morning time, then I've got one in! A good habit. Daily schedules can get confounded as our days lengthen – right? In my book of many lessons learned, a less-than-perfect session achieved is better than a perfect session missed.

Dan Pink offers primary benefits of afternoon workouts:

a. Injury avoidance
b. Timed top performances for endurance and strength
c. Enjoyment. You are awake, rather than a bit grumpy, grizzled, or groggy when you move metal or other objects, right? What if you need more satisfaction? *Do it 'til you're satisfied.*

When we were younger, perhaps as college athletes, two-a-day sessions were common. Question: What if I exercise for strength in the morning, then again after noon with complementary activity? Answer: Nowadays, some of us can and do adapt to the loading of two-a-day regimens. We proceed carefully and take the time needed to do our training right, and to recover. If you have the time and passion, go ahead and give twice-daily workouts a try. I can two or three daily workouts as an indoor rowing leader. Spice up your strength regimen occasionally. What you try—you may like.

You should also consider mixing up your activities or workout times for variety, and to learn about your unique circadian rhythms for strength, stamina, and sleep, as highlighted in other book chapters. Location, location, location?

Where?

Wherever. Anywhere, or nearly anywhere. It depends on you and your developing fitness habits.

Lift in your loft. Do bodyweight moves in your bedroom. Who said weights aren't fun? Certainly not Kama Sutra authors and practitioners. Gym workouts are fine, though some boomers feel intimidated by "all those contraptions" and grunting specimens or loud music. Don't be psyched out; particularly since our Medicare system allows "Silver Sneaker" athletes to join some gyms for free. Isn't America great? Note: As a former "big box" trainer, I assert that most fixed machines in corporate gyms offer poor returns for your KA-BOOMER strength work. I stated most, not all. Free weights and functional bodyweight training offer better returns—for wherever you lift, push, and pull stuff. And compound exercises generally beat isolated gym machine pumps. Trust me. Life isn't simple, so moving stuff shouldn't be simple either.

If you don't have weights in your plan of the day—due to travel or jail time—then body weight activities are fine for toning your muscles and maintaining what you've gained elsewhere. Youngish prisoners who lift for hours can build seriously buff muscle mass. Thankfully, most of you readers are not working out in striped pajamas and don't have the time to lift for hours! Having and using metal weights, resistance bands, and objects like battle ropes are great for your longevity and wellness. Anywhere you have body weight to move, you answer your own "where?"

Yes, Koach, but I just *don't* have time in my busy as heck Life to lift.

Try again! Try to convince your Koach that you can't. In other words, horsefeathers! I find time for what is important, and you need to find the time too—unless you decide it's just not important to you.

Quickie trivia: *Horsefeathers* was a 1932 Marx Brothers movie. These comedians were way ahead of Colin Kaepernick when they cast aspersions on football as a cultural sport, though they lagged Theodore Roosevelt who revamped "America's Game" in 1905. Strength is a critical part of America's Game, right? You too can find time, just as committed athletes do. If needed, bully! Revamp! Lift or move stuff quickly!

Example: A Tabata protocol can be completed in less than four minutes! After that interval session, your afterburn metabolism is revved, and you prove that being fast is good for some things, but not all things. Make the time for your four minutes.

Yes but, what if I was diagnosed with multiple sclerosis (MS)?
Yes but, I have rheumatoid arthritis. Should I toss in my towel and take it easy?
Yes but, I am troubled by asthma.
Yes but, I was diagnosed with adult diabetes.

So sorry but read on. My short and emphatic response to these Yes, buts (and any other excuses) is NO!

Experts remind us: **"Anyone, at any fitness level, can and should strength train. And it doesn't have to take hours at the gym to see results…. Grab a towel and get ready to feel strong."**[158]

Where is your towel? Now, how?

Here's How
With your towel and water bottle close at hand, start working those skeletal muscle groups (twice each week). Simple. Just get going. Then keep moving stuff.

Addendum D

Source Code for Strength

Question: What is the physical source of brandished human strength?

Answer: Little mice. Honest.

"Muscle" is "little mouse" in Latin. Sure, some of our 600+ muscle groups may be mouse-like in appearance. I hope that your muscles will evolve to be mighty mice. Your muscles and muscle groups are called sarcomeres by scientists.

How big are our sarcomeres (muscle fibers) as physical units for strength actions? It depends, though some are our body's biggest and longest cells with lengths up to 30 cm (or 11.8 inches) in our upper leg muscles. These fibers, which expand and contract in isotonic moves, are about 40 percent of our body mass (that is if we avert sarcopenia!). In case you want a deeper dive into muscle phenomena, call or contact me.... Just one twitchy point....

"Fast twitch" (Type I) fibers lose performance sooner than our "slow twitch" (Type II) muscle fibers as we blow out more candles. That's life. Hence, our sprint and anaerobic "burst" performance tends to degrade faster as we age than does our sustained endurance capacity. Stamininety isn't about sprinting! It is about superior performance in contrast to normal boomers.

Two of my favorite music types are Country and Western. I gotta modify Toby Keith's phrase: "I'm as good once as I ever was...." That isn't quite so for strength, but c'est la vie. My Keith-counter?

Our KABOOMER goal is to lose strength and power more slowly than others in our generation do.

Do not concede to aging and withering until you must. Keep your gym-age years much lower than that of your peers. Move stuff as your cornerstone of a physical 401(k). Let's consider the property value of your mighty mice.

What are valued properties or functions of skeletal muscles (sarcomeres)?

They: 1. excite, 2. contract, 3. extend, and 4. elastically re-coil.[159] Biochemistry is at work here, so I'll skip the darn for-mulaic details. Check my web blog posts or seminars to learn more about the biochemistry of strength. Don't be too con-cerned *if you don't know a pyruvate from a pear, or whether lactate is a smoothie drink or an energy source.* Just celebrate those biochemical reactions that have evolved over centuries and that happen every time, all the time, that you are moving.

There is much more to appreciate about our human strength system. Our amazing bodies can withstand blood pressures of approximately 350 mm/Hg over 150 mm/Hg in the peak phase of a relatively heavy lift or resistance move that we make. *Please check with your doctor to ensure that your cardiovascular system is ready to be challenged with loading transients like blood pressure.* My physician and my body allow me to move heavy weights, though I'm not always *brandishing* them. Our mind-body linkage is also fascinating. Our neurons are programmed for safety/survival in a throttle or regulator way:

"Your body is hardwired with a massive overabundance of reflexive and unconscious mechanisms to protect your body from physical damage."[160]

Sarcomere size counts in our strength, surely. But a more important factor is usually how many fibers our central ner-vous system (CNS) allows to trigger at one time. Most peo-ple cannot get their throttling nervous system to fire more than 30 percent of their available muscle fibers at one time. Elite athletes can respond with about 50 percent of their avail-able muscle factors via better recruitment and conditioning.

Why the throttle? Unregulated strength would be dangerous to our skeletal joints. Thus our CNS knows how to govern, throttle or regulate muscular work in a preventative sense. Such is life. Now, *let's work that 30 to 50 percent as best we can, as fast as we can, or for as long as we can.* These efforts are great ways to add longevity and quality of life. Period.

Work your muscles and joints (even if creaky or degraded) in *all three* of your body planes to balance efforts and to prevent imbalances. Recall that we can lift, move stuff or do resistance training in three ways: 1. fast, 2. heavy, and 3. long. What categories or types of strength make that stuff move? Here they are:

Four—Count Them—Four Types of KABOOMER Strength

We, like athletes of other age demographics, can show their FORTIUS with: 1. absolute, 2. dynamic, 3. elastic, and 4. endured strength efforts. Let's count 'em and then try 'em often....

1. **Absolute** strength is a demonstration of one's maximum force, irrespective of time. The world record deadlift is a "mere" 1,155 pounds (524kg) of dead weight. Lifting over half an English ton of stuff to one's waist level is one herculean load, which couldn't be accomplished without absolute strength.

   Note: Your starting load could be a five-pound bag of flour, or an overnighter suitcase, rather than a half-ton truck. Remember, you're not record holder Zydrunas Savickas or a brobdingnagian Captain America. You start with a dead weight that you can handle safely, then progress to heavier objects. No hysteria there, but over here....

   We also classify "hysterical" rescues as matters of absolute strength. We are fascinated by Herculean hoists!

One example: A special Samaritan, Tom Boyle, raised a Chevy Camaro high enough to save a person trapped underneath it, (under very special circumstances) as the BBC reported. (www.bbc.com/future/story/20160501-how-its-possible-for-an-ordinary-person-to-lift-a-car). Tom was able to briefly override his CNS safety circuitry to go full throttle (absolutely) in his lifesaving lift. By the way, Tom was a very big and very strong dude, at the right place at the right time to be a momentary over-riding hero.

2. **Dynamic** strength is one's muscular power exerted in repeated motions. An example of dynamic strength might be Supreme Court Justice Ruth Bader Ginsburg's workouts.[161] Ladies and Gentlemen, if this 80-something cancer survivor can work on her dynamic strength, we "younger folks" should repeat power exertions as well! May your dynamic (interval) work please the court, Seneca, and you.

3. **Elastic** strength is force in which you exert *quickly over distance*. Did you see or hear about how high a professional athlete, J. J. Watt, can box jump? His 57-inch box leap as a 280-pound football player is truly *elastic*. J. J. is what one might label a physical "freak of nature," so I'm okay with my mortal plyometric strength. Plyometric literally means "more measure." Plyometric strength operationally for you and me means "activities that enable a muscle to reach maximal force in the shortest time possible."[162] Folks like #99, J. J. Watt, are elastically able to trigger "fast twitch" muscle sequences. The technical name for such a quick draw motion is a *stretch shortening cycle* or SSC. J. J. Watt has a very short SSC. I do *not*. Watch Olympic power lifters—men and women. Watch elite CrossFit competitions—men and women. Such outliers are blessed with elastic strength and short SSC's. Perhaps you are too.

My grandkids like the *Incredibles* movie characters, including an elastic-limbed Mom. Her SSC is awesome. Granted, these *impulsive* powers and heavy lifts in blinks of the eye can't be humanly repeated as dynamic strength for longer periods of work. We're not transformers, or cyborgs, after all. *Please take away that you can strive to be the best that you can be for your own elasticity (SSC).*

4. **Extended** (endured) work is the basis for our fourth category of human strength. Endured strength is a lengthy set of resisted movement(s) to withstand one's bodily fatigue. Personal trainer David Chu offers this operational meaning for endured strength: "It's being able to do something that takes significant strength for a very long time. That's very different from, say, working towards a max(imum) single squat rep(etition)."[163]

A farmhand's work during long harvesting days of fatiguing manual labor is endurance strength. A farmer's walk is a fine endured strength measure of "gym age" strength for men and women.[164] Gym age, you say? You betcha. Strive for the endured "gym age" strength of younger people because you can. One of the finest examples of KABOOMER endured strength is performing a single pull up for a one-minute period. Yup, take 30 seconds to pull yourself up with chin over the bar, then take 30 seconds in a very slow down motion to the well "hung" position. Gym strong. When you are ready for an ultimate pull up, that is. Not before.

• * Metabolic weight sessions are extensions of this constantly and slowly changing contraction of your prime movers. Try as few "reps" as possible in ninety seconds! Then move quickly to your next planned set. Granted, these "metabolic" regimens are fast and efficient. Call or write me if you'd like to know more about these very slow resistance series.

You'll please yourselves and me when you learn to love functional endured strength moves like farmer's walks. Your body, your spouse or significant other, and your grandkids will thank you for your endured strength.

Think of a master's cross-fitter, a boomer pentathlete, or a decathlete as an activity "master" or competitive master's athlete who uses multiple types of strength in his or her journey.

Develop all your absolute, dynamic, endured and elastic strengths.

Be KABOOMER strong—in all four of these ways.

Lift on for strength in the spirit of J.J. Watt, Tom Boyle, and Ruth Bader Ginsburg. I advocate lifting to perform well and feel good, which you will. But wait, there's a nice (no kidding) perk.

Strength moves define body shape (in pleasing ways). Mirrors, kids, drunks, and Lululemon tights do not lie! None of these would lie about your *buff, lower gym-age body*. Next, let's consider some specific muscle groups that we should keep active. Trust me that your strang 1. toes, 2. quadriceps-(quads), 3. hip flexors, 4. "core," 5. shoulders, and 6 neck region, will get you to those parties at 90.

1. **Metatarsals** (toes). No kidding, our great toes are outsized in relevance for strength (and stability). Simple toe raises and heel raises are strength moves to avoid face plants and broken bones. Work those tiny abductors and tendons in your feet that can help you stay upright.

2. **Quadriceps** (our biggest sarcomeres) are a *beast mode* strength group for daily lives worth living. Our longest tendon, the iliotibial tract (or IT band), which stretches from our outer hips to our knees, should be worked and also stretched. Think deadlifts, squats, lunges…. Size matters.

3. **Hip flexors.** There is one *lone* muscle group that links our upper and lower body halves—the "deep core" or psoas group. Our psoas must be worked to stabilize our spines (with help from many other core muscle groups) as they hip-flex. *Do* work your hip flexors (psoas) regularly, for reasons more than spinal stability. Think about that. Then read more about your deep core and psoas muscles in our Stability chapter. Open and flex your hips.

4. **Lumbar and thoracic spine regions of your core— LPHC** and **Back**. Back issues are much ado about *something*! I speak from firsthand knowledge. I also speak from many client encounters, as backs and midsections are often sources of their discomfort or pain. I encourage folks to be proactive to the CORE.

5. **Shoulder girdle (particularly your rotator cuff)**. I certainly have experienced my share of shoulder problems after bicycle spills and excess exercise.... Many have heard of, or sensed, frontal shoulder pain (around what is called a rotator cuff (or RC)). Are you one of them?

   The four (4) muscle groups that enable your shoulder rotation are hard to pronounce, spell correctly, and memorize – so the term "RC" suffices for our potentially troubled: 1. Supraspinatus, 2. Infraspinatus, 3. Teres Minor, and 4. Sub-scapularis muscles. Think of resistance bands, and preventative, endured strength efforts and stretches to avoid RC issues!

6. **Neck Region**. I'm not a betting man. If I was, I would wager "with the house" that most boomers either have, or will have, neck issues in the years ahead. Think of a ten-pound bowling ball perched on a long, linked chain. Now think about avoiding a gutter ball!

   I'm not a great spell-checker for Latin-named muscles of our neck region either. I thank innerbody[165] authors and artists for sparing me more typos with this instructive webpage summary...

"Neck muscles, including the Sternocleidomastoid and the Trapezius, are responsible for the gross motor movement in the muscular system of the head and neck. They move the head in every direction... control the flexion and extension of your head and neck..... Neck muscles contract to adjust the posture of the head throughout the course of a day and have some of the greatest endurance of any muscles in the body."

Or *not*, if they are weakened from excess screen time, poor sleep posture, underuse, or structural issues. Keep your neck in the strike zone. Wow—from little mice to bowling balls—one more time...

Move the thing or one you're with. How long and how well we might live is truly extended by resistance work with objects like bands, weights, heavy cans of peas, or bags of sugar or beans. Don't neglect bodyweight resistance activities. After all, that amazing hulk of yours is always with you.

Don't stop! Science suggests that **85 years** is a *nominal* aging point when muscle building capacity drops notably. Until that venerable time stamp (as currently asserted), build sinews and retain vigor.

My strength as medicine keeps my gym age lower than my peers. Your Koach can help you lower yours as well. Please take a few minutes to review the next addendum—you'll learn technicalities to help you move stuff.

Addendum E

Strength Science

Few are Biochemists or Kinesthetic experts. Yet all of us should appreciate our corpus of strength, force, power and energy. Here is your Strength Appreciation Day for brandishing weights with vigor. Be savvy about strength, power and energy, okay?

1. Strength is work or force exerted (in ways as just described).
   a. Strength is work done against, or with resistance.
2. Power is strength or force per a unit of time.
   a. Power is strength exerted for some measured span (inch, foot, meter) per a unit of time.
3. Energy is stored in our bodies, not the force produced by our bodies.
   a. I'm looking at a teaspoon of cane sugar. That little amount of sugar equates to 70 kilojoules of energy. That's about one minute of energy to power one's hard rowing or running or swimming. Or, that's headed for fat storage if you don't move something.

A 70-year old female athlete doesn't have to be "Charlene Atlas"; she just needs to (dead)lift something to lengthen and thicken many muscle groups. That something can be a great grandkid lifted from the floor, or a carry-on duffel for Amtrak or American Airlines (I picked those carriers at random). She lengthens and thickens muscle fibers after power phases. Work is moving something for a given distance. Power is moving that something for that distance quickly. Likewise, for Charles K. who doesn't have to be "Charles Atlas" for working strength, power and energy use.

The Greek word "*ergon*" means, as you may have guessed, "work." Indoor rowing machines are called ergometers. I resonate with ERGs, as you have read. Whole-body work of ERGing (with about 600 muscle groups) is supported by the central nervous system, and lungs, and cardiovascular piping, as our very own personal strength and power systems. As a rower, I offer this "ERG" chuckle (from Urban Dictionary) about strength, power and work.

The Ergometer

"...an awful torture machine that should be illegal under the Eighth Amendment, but that gets out of jail free under a *loophole* that it is '*fun*.' Commonly used in the regime of an evil dictator by the name of 'Coach' and his/her faithful servant, the 'coxswain.' Originally derived from the Greek word meaning 'to work,' which is what one does—very, very hard, for a long, long time."[166]

When you "Erg" or perform work over a given time, you generate *power*. How quickly your strength allows you to lift "x" foot-pounds per second is your generated power for that lift at that time. Five hundred and fifty foot-pounds per second equates to one horsepower (HP). Some of us can generate a horsepower for short periods.

Remember—lift heavy and fast to generate "higher" power.

Powerful Trivia

You can find, via Dr. Google searches, that a few indoor cyclists or indoor rowers, "wired" in series, can generate enough electrical power to heat a toaster for brief spells. Okay—Hoover Dam is a bit bigger generator of power than Mark Cavendish or Lance Armstrong ever was or could be cycling up the French Alps. (Small print: Armstrong is a cancer survivor as a testament to overcoming obstacles. Granted, he probably wasn't clean of performance-enhancing steroids. Yet he is an impressive specimen for generating horsepower.)

Olympic "snatch" lifts are perfect examples of powerful elastic strength. Extraordinary elastic strength was needed for a Georgian, Lasha Talakhadze, to power 220 kilograms (492 pounds) over his head as the "snatch" world record in 2017.

This feat of uber-elastic strength equates to at least **2,200 foot-pounds** per second of his lift. That is about **3,000 watts**, or **four horsepower**. Think about that as a modern "Four Horsemen" feat. Don't try to beat Lasha; just try to generate power, then give those muscular power utilities of yours a break to restore and repair. Know your body and its recovery patterns.

Enforce your habits of resistance training, diet, and rest.

You can get caught in a theoretical swamp if you seek the truest or latest and greatest theory for human muscle building. I did! Most experts do agree that stem cells play key roles in muscle hypertrophy. But describing these amazing cells (which can also turn into fatty cells) is above my pay grade. I'll stick with the practical message: "get ready to do some hard work and prepare for slow gains."

Hard work? To the point of causing micro-tears in your and my muscle fibers. The after-effects of these micro-tears and intended inflammation are post-activity muscle soreness.

Slow gains? Think of your strength journey in timeframes of weeks and months. There are not instant, radical, or breakthrough techniques to hasten our natural process for muscle growth and repair. However, our cytokine messengers enable response to exercise-induced inflammation quite quickly. Some improvements that you can see and feel may be noted in as few as six weeks. I personally count on eight weeks or two months of focused strength building gains. Try it yourself; and your acquaintances, your mirror, and your clothes will notice your bodily gains.

Yes, and...

Can you advance both your personal strength and your endurance levels in stride? Yes. Studies, and my personal journals, suggest that simultaneous improvements can be made in both of our physical 401(k)s: strength and stamina. The magnitude of these improvements is unique for each boomer in his or her journey, based on—guess what? Workloads, diet, and rest. Did I repeat myself? Now—can we absolutely maximize our strength and stamina in stride? Not really, yet I don't care much about this. I care about adding years to my life and life to my years.

Beating Charles Atlas or embarking on a delusional chase of absolute strength records isn't my game in life.

Hmmm... How often are skeletal muscles regenerated by our bodies (before cellular senescence or ultimate demise)?

Scientists report that one to two percent of our muscles' myonuclei are regenerated each week. Yup! Your skeletal muscles are totally replaced every few months. Now that is a wellness makeover! What may be fascinating—if you are interested in intra-cellular matters—is that exercise lengthens the telomeres in your cells' DNA strands. These lengthened telomeres theoretically lengthen the clip-off times of these DNA "shoelace caps" and (drumroll, please)—and lengthen the times between a cell's suspended animation (scientists call this senescence) or death. **Longevity and improved cellular health—meet longer telomeres lengthened by exercise**.

Amanda Macmillan, a TIME reporter, stated:
"Telomeres, the protein caps on the ends of human chromosomes, are markers of aging and overall health. Every time a cell replicates, a tiny bit of telomere is lost, so they get shorter with age. ...*people who exercised the most had significantly longer telomeres than those who were sedentary....* People who did vigorous exercise had telomeres that signaled about seven fewer years of biological aging, compared to people who did moderate levels of activity."[168]

Dwell on that. **Seven more years** to party. Twenty-five hundred extra sunrises and days of wonder.

I recall one report, some thirty years ago, that questioned the virtues of strenuous exercise. Why invest a couple of years of your *lifespan in exercise, when you may only live a few years longer?* I didn't buy that "zero sum" stance even then—and that was years before this exciting result for the merits of exercise. *Those longevity naysayers should have read what the stoic Seneca wrote millennia ago. Now for muscle magic, inside out....*

Your *"average"* skeletal muscle cell is loaded with 750 to 1,000 tiny power plants called mitochondria. These mitochondria are what convert little chemical compounds into contractions to work. Our muscles have more mitochondria than the average glandular cells in our bodies. More of these tiny power plants means easier lifts of heavy suitcases, more easily tossing your grandkids, or better performing activities of daily life. Take that fact to build your physical 401(k) account! *Can you spare a fortnight for Fortius?* A fortnight to better convert protein to energy. Just two weeks. Anyone who grasps timely return on investments can grasp that!

Okay, Koach. I get your points of mighty little mice and mitochondria magic. I grasp the relationship of strength, power, and energy to do work. Is there any age-related topic of flagging performance that we should acknowledge?

Yes, there is! I'll see something and say something for Mr. and Mrs. T(estosterone) in our final Strength sub-addendum.

Addendum F

Testosterone and Adam

See Something, Say Something

Hormones and blood flow impact our erogenous zones and our flagstaffs. If hormones called androgens fade with age or other situations, libidinous performance can also fade. Fatigue, stress, alcohol, smoking, high blood pressure, and obesity are also reasons for diminished blood flow to erogenous zones. Cutting to the chase, male menopause (or **andropause**) is no laughing matter. Androgen decline in aging males (a.k.a. ADAM) can be a quality of life or life decrement for KABOOMER males and others around them. What are declining symptoms of ADAM? Here are those danger signs:

Symptoms of Male Menopause or ADAM[169]

Adverse changes in physical appearance
Body fat gain, particularly abdominal weight gain
Loss of lean muscle tissue
Bone deterioration
Loss of hair
Wrinkling and drying of the skin
Fatigue
Poor sleep quality or insomnia
Decreased libido, possible erectile dysfunction (ED)
Hot flashes (yup), blushing, and sweating
Aches and pains
Mental functions decline
Reduced motivation/apathy
Nervousness, anxiety, and irritability
Memory lapses
Depression

Question: Can resistance or strength training favorably (and naturally) address andropause for men?

Answer: You bet, Red Rider.[170]

Hold this! "Testosterone and human growth hormone (HGH) levels can be increased through exercises, specifically heavy weightlifting and 'High Intensity Interval Training' (HIIT)... you might want to engage in these types of work-outs for greater virility. Weight and Resistance Training and HIIT are also great to counterbalance the increases in visceral body fat, and the loss of lean muscle mass and bone density. In addition, rest and a healthy diet are equally important when trying to naturally boost your testosterone levels."[171]

Ladies: Testosterone ("T") is **vital** for your skeletal muscles too.

Guys: If your T level is notably lower than published population-wide averages for your age bracket, you might consider proactive steps to bump up your T. Speaking as a Medicare-aged KABOOMER and Koach, I take 'au naturel' steps and make those lifts to avert andropause symptoms.

Takeaway? Resistance training (with diet and sleep) can offset andropause effects on us[172] ... Lift. Work. Sinews. Vigor. Viagra may not be necessary if you hit the weights, eat clean, and rest!

Addendum G

Elephant No. 1: Diets

Lengthy books abound for diets, all types of diets. And that abundance is also true for online searches for Keto(ketogenic), Paleo, Dash, and Mediterranean diets.

Your successful diets are lengthy lifestyle habits, rather than two-week wonders.

Most valid diets are low-carbohydrate, appropriate-fat regimens.

Circle back to a succinct Younger Next Year mantra of Crowley and Dodge: *"**Don't eat crap.**"* Find what enduring dietary habits for good eating sustain you. Find those that have the best prospects to help you live longer and live better. KABOOM.

Space doesn't allow a full discourse on inflammation, collagen, or Ph.D.-level microbiome details, though these elements of quality sustenance and healthy diet are important. I offer a trusty resource for two terms of interest:

a. Collagen: www.organicauthority.com/energetic-health/ your-complete-guide-to-the-best-collagen-supplements Good point! "Before adding any type of supplement to your diet, it's important to talk to your doctor or nutritionist."

b Inflammation and anti-inflammatory sustenance: www. webmd.com/arthritis/psoriatic-arthritis/psa-17/slide-show-psa-inflammation-foods Good point! Doctors don't always share the bad lifestyle news www.everydayhealth.com/news/10-things-your-doctor-wont-tell-you-about-metabolic-syndrome/

If you have a moment, please log on and search keywords for the most popular diets and the diets deemed to be most "effective" for 2019 (or for your most recent calendar year). Feel free to surf with Dr. Google, or Prof. Safari, or the web browser of your choice.

Once you've found these diet lists, please repeat after me: "IT DEPENDS." Why? Each of us is a different car or model—so each of our metabolic tune-ups should be unique, too. What fuels and works for a Tesla may not work for a Volkswagon.

Most of us sense that most diet regimens (rather than 'lifestyle fueling' as the Mediterranean diet is sometimes labeled) result in failure if the measure of success is keeping the *weight* or *fat off*. I advocate lifelong lifestyle "diets" rather than "x-day" wonder diets for this reason. You probably know, as I do, a Medifast peer who unfortunately reverted to his or her "before" body composition after a short-term fix. Oy. Folks, I assert that it's *not* just calories in and calories out at the dinner table or snack bar. Energy equations are favorably or adversely impacted by sleep, stress, and sustenance. How does your energy equation shape up?

Addendum H

Elephant No. 2: Gut Reaction

The keyword "gut" is more prevalent on my recent Internet searches than these terms: detox, belly fat, breakthrough diet, probiotics, and "America's Biggest Loser." You may get scores of daily online Gut Health ticklers, like I do. By the way, I do subscribe to many diet and sustenance related sites, like mayoclinic.org, Harvard Health, Dr. Weil, and Healthy Living. Sensational "fool me once" claims do not originate in these trusted sites. You know how they go... "here's a breakthrough program for your gut to make you mentally sharp." "Here's an ancient GI remedy that has your name on it. Just type your *PayPal* account or credit card number here, and you're one step closer to gut health!" Voila.

More important than these distractions or PT Barnum teasers: you and I should be very thankful if we avert some aging problems that are microbiome related, such as:

1. "Leaky gut" for skin irritation
2. Increased inflammation
3. Sleep problems and fatigue
4. Autoimmune responses
5. Food intolerances.

Our extraordinary "head to tail" piping system, with trillions (yup) of organisms in our gastrointestinal (GI) tract, is called a *microbiome* by experts. This dietary system is far more than a process of eat, digest, expel from head-to-tail. Our GI tract—from mouth through stomach to intestines and dumpster—and as supported by other glands and organs— may be a "master cylinder" for our daily efforts. Do we face a favorable or unfavorable in-body relationship with this master cylinder? Yes. Is weight loss or gain related to one's "gut" issues? Yes!! Is learning more facts about + and - gut issues important? You bet. Guts are big deals, fer sure.

What's a boomer to do, without stressing over this master cylinder? My suggestions, backed by reasonable sources start with eating foods that your microbiome "eats", like onions, leeks, garlic, bananas, and asparagus.[173] And...

- Consume both soluble and insoluble fiber in adequate quantities as part of your "good carb" macronutrients. Think beans, oats, leeks, asparagus (again).

- Try to eat fermented food or drink products of "high quality"—kombucha, raw sauerkraut, kimchi, miso, and yogurt (but watch their sugar levels).

- Eat foods that help us naturally increase our collagen levels (which drop notably as we age). Think wild salmon, carefully selected bone broths, mushrooms, and some "good" dairy products to probably slow down wrinkles and saggy, crepey skin.

More Guts

Our gut is so important that fecal transplants may be needed to favorably impact a sick person's "bad gut." No kiddin'. I once sat next to a smart, young internist from Maryland on an airline flight. He shared that he performed fecal transplants—with quite favorable patient results for healthier guts. As this doctor was so impressive, I'll highlight two wellness items that he shared:

1. A good balanced and clean diet may limit the need for probiotic supplements for most of us.

2. A young, healthy Dad, whom he treated, died from the flu at Disneyland. He did not get a flu shot that year.

My flight chat takeaways?

Be smart. Take an extra step to live long and prosper. Get help if you have danger signals related to your gut. Try some changes to your daily dietary habits to help you maintain: a strong immune system, heart health, brain health, improved mood, healthy sleep, and effective digestion; and it may help to prevent some cancers and autoimmune diseases (like arthritis).

There are lifestyle changes you can make to affect your gut health in very positive ways. (See www.healthline.com/health/gut-health.)

Gut Health and Leaky Gut

Why should leaky gut syndrome concern you? Recently leaky gut has been called a "danger signal for **autoimmune disease**." If you're wondering if you may be experiencing leaky gut, the first thing to do is assess your symptoms. Keep in mind that it's very common for people on a standard American diet to struggle with poor gut function and high levels of inflammation—but just because digestive issues and autoimmune conditions are common doesn't make them "normal."[174]

Enough shared, except that **stress** and **sleep** are closely inter-related with gut health or gut-induced inflammation conditions. Did your Koach mention that yoga can aid your diet effectiveness? Stay tuned so that you can feel great, inside out!

A Healthy Wrap

Eating clean betters your prospects to achieve stamininety; your brass ring on the carousel of living long and living well. Unlike cancer! Like about seven to 10 active and vibrant years longer than a median boomer will experience! How?

- Clean diets favorably affect our blood pressure levels and can avert hypertension. Experts commend a diet called DASH to do just that—au naturel.
- We can increase sensitivity to insulin and possibly avert type 2 adult diabetes.
- Clean diets trigger "good" hormone functions for weight control and conversely turn down or turn off hormone triggers for obesity.

- Dietary fiber (which does not have to taste like sawdust, by the way) can help most of us lessen the chance of colorectal cancers. Fiber, as you'll see, is a subset of "carb" macronutrients.
- Clean 80/20 diets support libido by ramping up testosterone naturally.
- Clean diets support our microbiome "gut" to *counter* bodily inflammation and what public health officials call "*metabolic* syndrome." Sounds menacing – yes?
- Clean diets keep "old age" appearances, like saggy skin, wrinkles, and thinning hair, from appearing or worsening.

Addendum I

Elephant No. 3: Metabolic Syndrome Like a Cancer

Clean eating considerations for our anti-aging fight can off-set metabolic syndrome (MetS) which lurks as an unhealthy cluster of conditions that hinders far too many! Millions of our demographic peers tragically have disorder in their court. (Metabolic is a fancy term for our body's normal functions.)

This new age medical term (coined in the 1980s) combines age-old abnormal problems which are worsening for too many!

Sufferers of metabolic syndrome are much more likely to fall victim to three of America's endemic health problems, namely *adult diabetes, strokes, and cardiovascular disease.* If a loved one, a friend, or you have three or more of these listed bodily symptoms, your Koach implores you to start eating clean and moving more—and please call your Doctor!

1. Large waist that measures at least 35 inches (89 centi-meters) for women and 40 inches (102 centimeters) for men. Remember your Koach's admonition to lower your waist-to-hip ratio.
2. High triglyceride level: 150 milligrams per deciliter (mg/dl), or higher.
3. Reduced "good" or HDL cholesterol: Less than 40 mg/dL (1.04 mmol/L) in men, or less than 50 mg/dL (1.3 mmol/L) in women, of high-density lipoprotein (HDL) cholesterol.
4. Increased blood pressure: 130/85 millimeters of mercu-ry (mm Hg) or higher.
5. Elevated fasting blood sugar: 100 mg/dL (5.6 mmol/L) or higher.[175]

As a demographic segment, baby boomers are at higher risk of hypertension because of age. Some of us (Mexican Americans) are more likely at risk because of heritage. Some of African American heritage may also be more prone to hypertension. All of us are at much higher risks if we carry too much weight (fat) around our midsections. Or smoke. Or sit too often as couch potatoes. Please pay attention to your midsection, and to the unclean foods that tempt you!

Addendum J

Fatty Elephant No. 4

Do not get *impressed* by the imposing and depressing Elephant No. 4 in our midst: Fat.

Fat that can sit right in our middle and persist *viscerally* around the organs in our midsection.

How *unfitting* are these lyrics from the Broadway play, Oliver (1986):

Food Glorious Food
Food, glorious food!
Eat right through the menu.
Just loosen your belt
Two inches and then you
Work up a new appetite.

Loosen my Belt?!

There is no finer manifesto about **fat** as a greatly misunderstood bodily organ (that's right an organ) than Sylvia Tara's *The Secret Life of Fat*. This healthy read should be on every KABOOMER's reading list. I offer this poignant image (below) to characterize one of our First World Problems, which Dr. Tara addresses.

Avoirdupois[176]

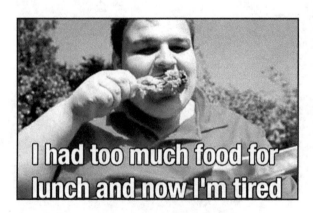

Is this pictured tubby teen over-eating in America's fattest city? Maybe yes, maybe no. Yet a person's zip code and economic status do relate with excess fat and unhealthy living. What was America's fattest city?

Mick Cornett, mayor of America's former fattest city, Oklahoma City, Oklahoma (OKC), might give you gas pains and then give you hope. OKC was first on a public wall of shame for hosting more fast food restaurants, per capita, than any other US city. Oy! Wait, wait, there is a silver lining! As a walk his talk role model, Mayor Cornett skipped over the river "De-Nile," and lost an average of one pound a week for forty weeks. That should be a sustainable goal: a pound (3,500 KCAL) a week of fat loss, which is just 500 dietary calories a day in his metabolic energy equation! He led social conversations and formed informal accountability steps for his citizens to record a loss of *1,000,000 pounds of fat*! I hope that most of these fatty pounds remained "off."

Yes, I over-simplified just a little about sustained fat loss, as our bodies adapt to our changing metabolism and may stubbornly stay on plateaus for a spell. Tweaking one's diet a bit and ramping up parts of one's regular workouts may help get past such plateaus. In some instances, "diet breaks" may aid your cause.[177]

Or, they may not. Prudence on your journey is advised, with a worldly reminder that "a body at rest tends to stay at rest." Borrowing (or abusing) this physical law of motion from Sir Isaac Newton, I suggest that outside forces (your shifts) are needed to goose one's metabolism off an "unsatisfactory" plateau, or a discouraging short-term lack of progress toward goals. Is all well outside OKC? Not really.

90210
Zip Codes matter for eating habits! Here's my short quiz for you:

Where did your county rank in our National Data for Obesity (for 2016)? [178, 179]

Condolences to any readers who live in Holmes County, Mississippi, because you were gauged to be *Numero Uno* (with a statistical 47 percent obesity rate for 2016).

Location, location, location

Recall the *less* healthy apple shape of too many adults. Recall the prevalence of waist to hip ratios that are "too high" for living longer and better.

Most Boomers, as in a majority of *75 million Americans* born between 1946 and 1964, carry extra and *unhealthy* fatty tissue, as defined by federal and refereed academic sources.[180] What is scary, is that much of this extra baggage reacts to become dreaded white, deep, and *lingering fat.* This is our pernicious, silent killer kind of fat. *Danger Will and Wilma Robinson.*

Your mirror and your clothes are darned good estimators of body fat (and skeletal muscle too). If you don't want to take the time to pinch your central fat, just see how your "8 pack" of abs looks. Ladies and gentlemen, if you can see your rectus abdominus muscles, you're probably not obese. We carry a lot of our boomer fat amidships. Four percent body fat is considered the minimally healthy level, as our body's essential functions and organs need fat!

Recall three categories of strength in an alternate chapter: a. decent; b. good enough; and c. excellent. Here, in the following Table, are relative, measured body fat percentages for these three breakouts for female and male boomers by age. Sure—you can be skinny but not strong. Sure, you can be overweight yet still perform well. *What is most important for this linkage of strength and body fat is your personal want and need.* Guys, we can't all be Hugh Jackman. Yet we can strive to be a bit leaner and stronger until we're 90 years young or more. Ladies, ditto. Unless we are sumo wrestlers, lean body types tend to live better and are generally more athletic. Unless we want to shorten our lives, we shouldn't get too plump. Strive for pears and lower WTHRs! We need "some" fat, yet we need it in "all the right places."

Reasonable Body Fat Percentages for Boomer Category of Strength and Stamina

Strength/ Stamina Categories	Range of measured Body Fat (Female)	Boomer Age Bracket (Female)	Range of measured Body Fat (Male)	Boomer Age Bracket (Male)
Decent	29 31 33	< 50 – 60 age 61-70 age 71 > age	24 26 28	< 50 – 60 age 61-70 age 71 > age
Good Enough	20 25 27	< 50 – 60 age 61-70 age 71 > age	18 20 22	< 50 – 60 age 61-70 age 71 > age
Excellent	< = 17 20 23	< 50 – 60 age 61-70 age 71 > age	< = 12 15 18	< 50 – 60 age 61-70 age 71 > age

One's body fat (BF) trend, gauged on the same device over time, or via indirect methods (look in the mirror, or gauge how your clothes fit) is more important than an absolute one-time value of BF. Wanna make lean happen?

I believe it was Robert Kennedy who cited three classes of people: 1. those who watch things happen; 2. those who ask, "what happened?"; and 3. those people who *make things happen.*

Do your habitual best to *make things happen.* Yes, you can. Guys, you can favorably change your WTHR. Ladies, you can say sayonara to most of your "muffin tops." Has it really been about 40 years since George Lucas released his first block-buster in 1977? Seems to me that a classic comment by that Jedi fitness mentor, Yoda, fits: "Do, or Do Not. There is No try."

Kudos, little green guy. Kudos to us who *do* make things happen. Make extra fat around your midsection shrink!

As many of my personal trainer clients share, and as suggested by informal pulsing of our generational members, body composition is important to us. It's not just appearance. It is that, plus their and our longer and better lives.

Way down our journeyed roads, when our partying slows a bit, we future nonagenarians and centenarians may benefit from stored "healthier than white" brown fat (read Dr. Tara's excellent book for more). Till then, we will keep up skeletal muscle mass, and therefore, our relatively high metabolism and physical capacity, for as long as naturally possible. In your scribe's current case, that means about *two more decades* of work and play (with weights and resistance training) to fend off sarcopenia and keep my pear shape and low waist to hip ratio (WHR). Skeletal muscle up, visceral fat down. Clean eating enables that transition. KABOOM.

I offer what I've found to be an *effective* way to plan/use daily sustenance for my body composition and vitality. Note: There is nothing, absolutely nothing, wrong with your counting of calories, or using smart phone/watch fitness tracker applications. Or following a formal diet, possibly under the watchful eye of a nutritional pro or medical doctor. I don't—but you may.

Setting a KABOOMER Example
What do I do, hopefully as an example to my clients and readers, to get the macronutrients I need for my KABOOMER lifestyle?

First, I strive to eat more than 30 grams of complete protein, and five or more grams of fiber when I eat my main meals.

And I drink plenty of clean water before I'm thirsty and with every meal or snack.

I strive to eat these daily totals as a ratio of my current body weight. And you can too...HINT.

Macronutrient Goals for KABOOMERs		
Macronutrient	Daily Amount	Gender
High protein	One gram per pound of current body weight	Both male and female
Enough "good" fat Low overall	One half gram per pound of body weight	Both male and female
Carbohydrates	100 total grams (including fiber)	Male
	50 grams (including fiber)	Female

Note the single variant for gender above: Carbohydrates. Men are generally heavier and bigger than women. We can eat "more" healthy carbs to fuel our muscles and help move food through our gut....

Fix Your Hormones

Not all carried fat is "our fault." No foul, no guilt. Just a fact.

My family has a documented fat gene. My siblings are more endomorphs than mesomorphs. None of my kin are ectomorphic "skinnies."

Sure, other families stay thin, as ectomorph body types, regardless if they eat blubber.

I'm not looking to fault fat. We should be mindful of our unique chemical messaging, which definitely and dramatically affects "fat burning," metabolic rates, and body composition.

An amazing regulator in our amazing bodies is our endocrine system, including our thyroid gland, our pea-sized yet masterful pituitary glands, and gonads too.

Do this mindful and healthful check on a pair of growth regulators that our master gland (pituitary) secretes—Growth Hormone (GH) and IGF-1 (officially named Insulin-like growth factor 1).[181] These are profoundly good chemical messengers for stamininety. And diet profoundly influences both!

Dr. Johnny Bowden helps us assess our endocrinal messaging and fat metabolism with five questions:[182]

Ladies and gentlemen, do you...

1. **Have more than an inch of body fat** stored on your right love handle? If you can pinch more than the length of your index finger's second joint, answer **YES**.
2. **Feel sleepy after eating a rich meal**, especially one hour after eating a "carb"-heavy lunch? If so, answer **YES**.
3. **Currently carry more than 30 pounds** of extra weight that you've tried to lose at least three times without success? If so, answer **YES**.
4. **Have cellulite or other areas of pocket obesity**, such as a lower belly pouch, or "saddle bags" on the hips and thighs? If so, answer **YES**.
5. **Struggle with losing weight and keeping it off**, even when restricting calories or going on an exercise plan? If so, answer **YES**.

If you answered yes to 2 or more of the questions above, your Insulin Growth Factor, a.k.a. IGF-1,[183] messaging may need a tune-up.

What about me? Dr. Bowden's quiz result suggests that I don't need his rev-up, at least not now. I'm reasonably blessed by nature, and I have worked to keep my metabolic hormones working at tuned-up levels. Do you sense or know that you're borderline for IGF-1, or leptin,[184] or dicey for our hunger hormone, ghrelin?[185] If so, all the fasting and exercise in our world may not get you to the body fat level, or healthy waist to hip ratio, that you want or need! As Dr. Bowden reinforces, "It's **not** your fault."

There are indeed lifestyle "pathways" to help us get closer to healthier pear silhouettes and partying performance, with tuned up chemical messaging. Get it done. KABOOM.

Recall item six from Fitzgerald's performance process, which I offered earlier in a main chapter:

Reducing cortisol (the stress or fight/flight messenger). If one's episodic or chronic stress is "too high" for "too long," survival instincts wired into our reptilian brains goose up our fat storage – rather than bumping up our fat-burning furnaces.

Clean eating steps and sustained dietary habits can support our body's vital, metabolically active tissues[186] (MATs). Think of heart, lung, kidney, muscle, and you have found MATs. MATs are sensitive to ebbs and flows of our endocrinal switch messengers—like leptin, cortisol, ghrelin, insulin, IGF-1, and other enzymes or hormones. As we age, these chemical switches can get wobbly or get stuck. Don't allow that, or work to get these switches unstuck. And, as a MAT lowlight, our fat (a.k.a. adipose tissue) is an organ that is constantly active too (according to Dr. Tara's The Secret Life of Fat). We can and should appreciate just enough chemistry to learn how to shrink our fat cells, so we can live better and longer. Trust Women's Health[187] (guys too!):

"Hormones dictate what your body does with food. **Fix your hormones and your body will slim down.**"

Virginia Slimmers, are you game for your tune-ups? **Fix 'em.**

Tune Up Masters

Hormone messengers (those chemical catalysts) largely determine whether we convert ingested calories to stored energy (fat) or metabolize it to move, to sleep or to digest food. *What* most of us boomers eat, plus *when* we eat, can help rev up latent "teenage/hollow leg/eat anything" metabolisms. Yes, some of us may have nature working against us, yet dietary tune-ups are cited for your possible consideration.

Note *fat-burning* as a theme. We all are capable of fat-burning to varying degrees. Are you highly effective as a natural fat burner? If so, your vital waist ratios for height and hips are likely to be strong markers for health and longevity.

Or do your stem cells create fat cells particularly in pockets, on your love handles or belly? If so, it likely isn't your natured fault that you are a poor fat burner. Perhaps you were when younger or perhaps not. Let's look ahead, not backwards. My waist is an inch bigger now than it was when I was 40 years old, although my overall body fat is about the same. Some of you may have been "there" at some time in your earthly journey or are "there" now. Remember, don't look back; act forward. Minimize unhealthy and central/visceral fat. Period.

Hacks to Burn Better

Most folks in the "poor" categories of fat storage vs. effective fat burning can do better. How? Start by skipping the French fries (because of their bad fat type) and remember good ol' *portion sizes.* Tweak your enzymes and hormones like a teen does. And/or tweak your messengers like an adaptive fat burner must – with a 'lil bit extra effort on your journey. General and affordable natural steps to "fat-burn" are:

- Pop plenty of plant-based flavonoids such as quality green tea.
- Naturally clean your liver with oleic acid foods (mostly plants like avocados).

- Tune your exercise routines (with professional help if merited).
- Be active with stress reducing efforts, and
- Be super-duper with good ol' deep Z's.
- Time your remedial actions for best effect.
- Try intermittent fasting. I do and not just because Hugh Jackman does.

We can eat clean to limit body fat and help our hormones. As we age, those glands are flashing SOS. We can listen and then answer the call for help.

It is true that the closer your KABOOMER efforts get you to your desired fitness and wellness goals, the harder it may be to continue or to reach for your next brass ring. Lean, healthy people find it harder to lose fatty weight, because they have less fat than America's Biggest Losers do, right? That's what nature has given us. As our body's metabolic systems improve, it is a 'lil bit harder to improve. Darn. Remember, it's a wellness journey with great returns on your natural investments. Give yourself a combo *nature and nurture* hug if you're working on your last one to two pounds of belly fat and offsetting occasional hunger pangs.

KABOOM. Thrive. Strive. KABOOM into your 90s.

Endnotes

Introduction and Chapter 1

1. https://www.ncbi.nlm.nih.gov/pmc/articles/PMC3555024/

2. https://www.psychologytoday.com/us/blog/the-resilient-brain/201704/restorative-sleep-is-vital-brain-health

3. https://www.cancer.gov/about-cancer/causes-prevention/risk/obesity/physical-activity-fact-sheet

4. http://www.fitdigits.com/phone/why-personal-heart-rate-zones.html

5. https://www.verywellfit.com/karvonen-formula-1229753

6. https://www.ncbi.nlm.nih.gov/pmc/articles/PMC6284760

7. https://well.blogs.nytimes.com/2014/10/15/whats-your-fitness-age/

8. https://www.apa.org/monitor/2017/10/cover-sleep

Chapter 2

9. https://www.ncbi.nlm.nih.gov/pmc/articles/PMC3312397/

10. https://www.ted.com/talks/wendy_suzuki_the_brain_changing_benefits_of_exercise/transcript?language=en

11. https://www.wsj.com/articles/astronauts-can-with-stand-longer-space-trips-new-study-of-twins-finds-11555005600?mod=searchresults&page=1&pos=1

12. https://dothemath.ucsd.edu/2013/12/a-physics-based-diet-plan/

13. https://experiencelife.com/article/everything-you-always-wanted-to-know-about-sweat/

14. Alex Hutchinson, *Endure Mind, Body and the Curiously Elastic Limits of Human Performance.*

15. http://sourcesofinsight.com/the-new-science-aging/

16. https://www.menshealth.com/fitness/a25169323/fitness-age-test/

17. https://www.worldfitnesslevel.org/

18. https://www.whyiexercise.com/VO2-Max.html

19. https://www.bluezones.com/live-longer-better/

20. https://www.nextavenue.org/key-longevity-health-biore-silience/

21. https://www.mayoclinic.org/diseases-conditions/metabolic-syndrome/symptoms-causes/syc-20351916

22. https://enduranceworks.com/blog/tips-for-the-masters-triathlete-40-years-old/

23. https://www.thedailymeal.com/healthy-eating/beer-athletes-post-workout-snack-you-always-wanted/111417

24. https://us.humankinetics.com/blogs/excerpt/dehydration-and-its-effects-on-performance

25. https://us.humankinetics.com/blogs/excerpt/how-periodization-is-used-by-endurance-athletes

26. https://tim.blog/2015/12/22/amelia-boone/

27. Chris Bergland, *The Athlete's Way: Sweat and the Biology of Bliss.*

28. https://vimeo.com/232565071

29. https://www.washingtonpost.com/national/health-sci-

ence/marathon-runners-who-drink-too-much-water-are-at-risk-of-a-deadly-condition/2011/10/10/gIQA-3imSDM_story.html

30.   http://www.endofthreefitness.com/murphys-law-fitness-edition-can-you-be-better/

31. https://www.spinemd.com/news-philanthropy/leg-length-discrepancy-linked-to-lower-back-pain

Chapter 3

32. https://www.semanticscholar.org/paper/Resistance-training-is-medicine%3A-effects-of-on-Westcott/2984736da22b5508a2d1d9cba7488b039097d2cc

33. https://www.exrx.net/Calculators/HealthAge

34. https://www.strategicamerica.com/blog/2012/10/just-the-facts-maam/

35. https://www.sciencedirect.com/science/article/abs/pii/S0167494318301493

36. https://perform-360.com/science-bulky-difference-bodybuilding-strength-training-physique/

37. https://www.wikihow.fitness/Measure-Muscular-Strength

38. https://www.verywellhealth.com/activities-to-avoid-after-total-hip-replacement-2696463

39. https://modernstoicism.com/show-me-your-shoulders-the-stoic-workout/.

40. https://dailyburn.com/life/fitness/how-to-build-muscle-fast-pick-weights/

41. https://www.verywellfit.com/muscle-hypertrophy-definition-3120349

42. https://health.usnews.com/wellness/fitness/articles/2018-03-23/11-benefits-of-strength-training-that-have-nothing-to-do-with-muscle-size

43. https://www.reuters.com/article/us-health-grip-strength/strong-grip-may-predict-longer-life-at-all-ages-idUSKCN1IM1TA

44. https://physicalculturestudy.com/2017/05/26/the-somewhat-complete-history-of-the-deadlift/

45. https://www.nfpt.com/blog/how-to-do-deadlift-with-a-bar-2

46. https://medicine.academic.ru/22011/ergogenic

47. https://www.drugabuse.gov/publications/drugfacts/anabolic-steroids

48. https://www.ncbi.nlm.nih.gov/m/pubmed/10079702/

49. https://www.ncbi.nlm.nih.gov/pmc/articles/PMC4269139

50. www.webmd.com/pain-management/guide/quality-of-life-scale-for-pain

51. https://www.theguardian.com/lifeandstyle/2013/mar/25/tabata-harder-faster-fitter-quicker

52. https://geriatrictoolkit.missouri.edu/balance/Normative_Values_for_the_Unipedal_Stance_Test_Springer-JGPT.pdf

53. https://www.thealternativedaily.com/if-you-balance-one-leg-might-mean-this/

54. https://www.prevention.com/fitness/fitness-tips/a20440531/the-stand-sit-test-that-predicts-longevity/

55. https://www.cdc.gov/steadi/pdf/STEADI-Assessment-30Sec-508.pdf

56. https://www.youtube.com/watch?v=oQIbffQj2xM

57. https://www.physiology.org/doi/full/10.1152/physrev.00048.2011#

58. https://www.silversneakers.com/blog/balance-stability-exercises-seniors/

59. https://journals.lww.com/topicsingeriatricrehabilitation/Abstract/2014/01000/ Qi_Gong_to_Improve_Postural_Stability__QTIPS__for.8.aspx

60. https://www.everydayhealth.com/multiple-sclerosis/living-with/best-exercises-boost-wellness-with-multiple-sclerosis/#wall-squats-strength-training

61. https://www.thealternativedaily.com/if-you-balance-one-leg-might-mean-this/

62. https://seniorsforseniors.ca/best-exercises-to-help-seniors-maintain-their-balance

63. https://www.verywellfit.com/how-stretching-can-help-you-lose-weight-3495386?utm_source=emailshare&utm_medium=social&utm_campaign=mobilesharebutton2

64. https://www.nfpt.com/blog/interpreting-signs-of-overhead-squat-assessment-lumbo-pelvic-hip-complex-dysfunction

65. https://rowingstronger.com/2016/07/11/fixing-rowing-imbalances/#more-3777

66. https://rowingstronger.com/2016/07/11/fixing-rowing-imbalances/#more-3777

67. https://www.nfpt.com/blog/why-the-psoas-is-significant

68. http://www.berkeleywellness.com/fitness/injury-prevention/article/get-know-your-psoas-muscles

69. http://coreawareness.com

Chapter 5

70. https://www.recoverfrominjury.com/

71. https://www.wholelifechallenge.com/stretch-bother/

72. https://www.verywellfit.com/exercise-for-beginners-why-flexibility-is-so-important-1229579

73. https://www.cdc.gov/arthritis/basics/osteoarthritis.htm

74. https://www.refinery29.com/en-us/worlds-greatest-stretch

75. https://www.silversneakers.com/blog/stretching-for-seniors-7-simple-moves-for-the-not-so-flexible/

76. https://www.verywellfit.com/shoulder-flexibility-test-3120278

77. https://www.livestrong.com/article/415584-what-exercise-should-i-do-if-i-cant-put-my-arms-behind-my-back/

78. https://www.silversneakers.com/blog/stretching-for-seniors-7-simple-moves-for-the-not-so-flexible/

79. https://www.nfpt.com/blog/knee-anatomy-structure-and-injuries

80. https://www.runnersworld.com/plantar-fasciitis/

81. Todd Hargrove, *Playing with Movement.*

82. https://www.bettermovement.org/blog/2019/the-new-book-is-here-playing-with-movement

83. https://www.health.com/fitness/dynamic-warmup

84. https://www.spine-health.com/glossary/myofascial-release

85. https://www.nfpt.com/blog/improve-client-flexibility-yoga-series

86. https://www.nfpt.com/blog/everything-you-need-to-know-about-sleep-fitness

87. https://www.drnorthrup.com/psoas-muscle-vital-muscle-body/

88. https://www.strengthandconditioningresearch.com/foam-rolling-self-myofascial-release/

89. https://www.spartascience.com/resources/closed-chain-exercise-is-crucial

Chapter 6

90. https://www.etymonline.com/word/stress

91. https://medical-dictionary.thefreedictionary.com/cortisol

92. https://www.latimes.com/home/la-hm-erskine-column-20181211-story.html

93. https://www.buildinglearningpower.com/2015/11/sorting-out-resilience-perseverance-and-grit/

94. https://www.youtube.com/watch?v=pxBQLFLei70

95. https://www.scientificamerican.com/article/what-happens-in-the-brain-during-sleep1/

96. https://chrissajnog.com/combat-mindset/

97. https://youtu.be/aT-r3-I6eY0

98. https://wellness.pittsburghsymphony.org/can-you-fight-stress-with-music/

99. https://www.inc.com/justin-bariso/want-to-increase-your-emotional-intelligence-watch-these-5-ted-talks-to-day.html.

100. https://www.psychologytoday.com/us/blog/the-athletes-way/201301/cortisol-why-the-stress-hormone-is-public-enemy-no-1 and https://www.webmd.com/balance/guide/blissing-out-10-relaxation-techniques-reduce-stress-spot#1

101. https://www.sleepfoundation.org/how-sleep-works/what-happens-when-you-sleep

102. https://www.howsleepworks.com/what_definition.html

103. https://www.psychologytoday.com/us/blog/the-resilient-brain/201704/restorative-sleep-is-vital-brain-health

104. https://www.nhlbi.nih.gov/files/docs/public/sleep/healthy_sleep.pdf

105. http://sitn.hms.harvard.edu/flash/2018/clearing-junk-healthy-lifestyle-choices-boost-brain-waste-disposal/

106. https://www.medicalnewstoday.com/kc/serotonin-facts-232248

107. https://www.hopkinsmedicine.org/health/wellness-and-prevention/low-sex-drive-could-it-be-a-sign-of-depression

108. https://www.nytimes.com/2012/10/18/booming/baby-boomers-and-insomnia.html

109. Dan Pink, When: The Scientific Secrets of Perfect Timing.

110. https://www.inverse.com/article/41171-best-sleep-apps

111. https://www.medicalnewstoday.com/articles/317816.php

112. http://www.saragottfriedmd.com/six-tips-for-better-sleep-improved-detoxification-and-weight-loss/

113. https://www.foodmatters.com/article/not-sleeping-it-could-be-your-gut-health

114. https:/www.nytimes.com/2011/03/05/health/05patient.html

115. Tim Ferriss, *Tools of Titans: The Tactics, Routines, and Habits of Billionaires.*

116. https://sciencebasedmedicine.org/melatonin-for-sleep-disorders-safe-and-effective/

117. https://www.webmd.com/heart-disease/resveratrol-supplements

118. https://www.sleepscore.com/how-a-nightcap-can-ruin-your-sleep/

119. https://www.healthline.com/nutrition/19-best-prebiotic-foods

120. https://www.nfpt.com/blog/is-your-epoc-epic-understanding-the-bodys-oxygen-debt

121. https://www.theguardian.com/sport/2003/jun/01/athletics.features2

122. https://www.afpafitness.com/research-articles/muscle-recovery-from-extreme-endurance-events

Chapter 7

123. https://www.theverge.com/2015/2/9/8003971/low-fat-dietary-health-goals-bad-science

124. https://www.cancer.org/cancer/cancer-causes/diet-physical-activity/diet-and-physical-activity.html

125. https://www.healthline.com/health-news/aging-actor-james-gandolfini-had-risk-factors-for-heart-attack-062113#1

126. https://www.heart.org/en/health-topics/heart-attack/life-after-a-heart-attack/lifestyle-changes-for-heart-attack-prevention

127. https://www.mayoclinic.org/diseases-conditions/metabolic-syndrome/symptoms-causes/syc-20351916

128. https://www.ncbi.nlm.nih.gov/pubmed/19335941

129. https://www.economist.com/node/21699184/comments

130. https://nutritionfacts.org/healthkit/

131. https://blog.aicr.org/2018/12/31/2018-a-year-of-defining-diet-quality/

132. https://www.menshealth.com/fitness/a28916177/arnold-schwarzenegger-terminator-diet-workout/

133. https://www.linkedin.com/pulse/6-rules-success-arnold-schwarzenegger-mohammad-rashid/

134. https://www.healthline.com/nutrition/how-much-protein-per-day

135. https://www.mayoclinic.org/healthy-lifestyle/nutrition-and-healthy-eating/expert-answers/clean-eating/faq-20336262

136. https://www.ted.com/talks/dan_buettner_how_to_live_to_be_100

137. https://www.ncbi.nlm.nih.gov/pubmed/12468415

138. https://www.todaysdietitian.com/newarchives/td_020909p40.shtml

139. https://www.todaysdietitian.com/newarchives/td_020909p40.shtml

140. https://www.mayoclinic.org/healthy-lifestyle/weight-loss/in-depth/metabolism/art-20046508

141. https://www.health.harvard.edu/staying-healthy/micronutrients-have-major-impact-on-health

142. https://www.webmd.com/healthy-aging/news/20121130/older-adults-vitamins-supplements#1

143. https://www.health.harvard.edu/staying-healthy/add-color-to-your-diet-for-good-nutrition

144. https://www.scientificamerican.com/article/the-messy-facts-about-diet-and-inflammation/

145. http://www.eatingforenergy.com/baby-boomers-and-vitamin-supplements/

146. https://www.besthealthmag.ca/best-eats/nutrition/nutrition-the-health-benefits-of-citrus-peels/

147. https://greatist.com/health/reasons-to-drink-water

148. https://www.beaumont.org/health-wellness/blogs/know-the-difference-between-heat-stroke-heat-exhaustion

149. https://www.mayoclinic.org/diseases-conditions/metabolic-syndrome/symptoms-causes/syc-20351916

150. https://www.ncbi.nlm.nih.gov/pmc/articles/PMC5044938/

151. https://www.bluezones.com/2018/08/best-foods-to-eat-to-reverse-the-deadly-effects-of-air-pollution/

152. https://www.ncbi.nlm.nih.gov/pub-med/11032452

Chapter 9

153. http://www.greatexpectations.org/wp-content/uploads/pdf/lp/responsibility/Responsibility%20poems.pdf

154. https://www.npr.org/templates/transcript/transcript.php?storyId=481291161

Addenda

155. https://www.health.harvard.edu/exercise-and-fitness/7-tips-for-a-safe-and-successful-strength-training-program

156. https://www.physio-pedia.com/home/

157. Daniel Pink, *When: The Scientific Secrets of Perfect Timing.*

158. https://www.nytimes.com/guides/well/strength-training-plyometrics

159. https://sciencing.com/four-properties-muscle-cells-22946.html#socialshare

160. https://www.bettermovement.org/blog/2008/the-central-nervous-system

161. https://abcnews.go.com/Health/Wellness/workout-supreme-court-justice-ruth-bader-ginsburg/story?id=50546669

162. https://athletics.fandom.com/wiki/Plyometrics

163. https://www.quora.com/What-is-strength-endurance

164. https://www.menshealth.com/fitness/a25169323/fitness-age-test/

165. https://www.innerbody.com/anatomy/muscular/head-neck

166. https://www.urbandictionary.com/define.php?term=erg

167. https://www.youtube.com/watch?v=fCwYhpT4cvE

168. http://time.com/4776345/exercise-aging-telomeres/

169. http://www.antiagingatlanta.com/menopauseandropause001.htm

170. http://www.backinform.com/the-influence-of-exercising-on-andropause-aka-male-menopause/

171. http://www.backinform.com/the-influence-of-exercising-on-andropause-aka-male-menopause/__

172. Ref: 8/26/2017 *Strength Training Past 50*-3rd Edition:

173. http://www.humankinetics.com/excerpts/excerpts/13-reasons-for-engaging-in-resistance-training2/2

    https://www.healthline.com/nutrition/19-best-prebiotic-foods

174. https://draxe.com/7-signs-symptoms-you-have-leaky-gut/

175. https://www.mayoclinic.org/diseases-conditions/metabolic-syndrome/diagnosis-treatment/drc-

20351921

176. https://antiimperialism.files.wordpress.com/2012/10/first_world_problems_3.jpg

177. http://www.ideafit.com/fitness-library/study-taking-breaks-from-dieting-can-boost-weight-loss

178. http://www.countyhealthrankings.org/explore-health-rankings/rankings-data

179. https://www.usnews.com/news/slideshows/study-the-worst-us-counties-for-your-health?slide=2

180. https://www.niddk.nih.gov/health-information/health-statistics/overweight-obesity

181. https://www.health.harvard.edu/diseases-and-conditions/growth-hormone-athletic-performance-and-aging

182.   http://leanmuscularbody.com/metabolic-factor-review/

183. https://www.ncbi.nlm.nih.gov/pmc/articles/PMC1187088/

184. https://www.webmd.com/diet/obesity/features/the-facts-on-leptin-faq

185. https://www.yourhormones.info/hormones/ghrelin/

186. https://www.healthstatus.com/health_blog/wellness/how-to-naturally-turn-your-slow-metabolism-into-a-fast-fat-burning-machine/

187. https://www.womenshealthmag.com/weight-loss/a19949845/turn-off-hormones-for-weight-loss/

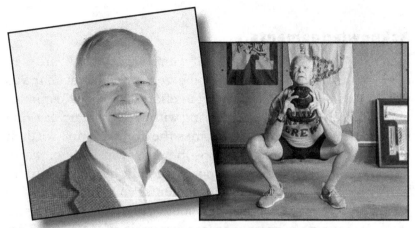

On any day which ends in a "y", KABOOMER Koach Dave Frost can be found training others, teaching learners of all ages, or doing charitable work for both wounded warriors and under-served youth. You may learn of healthy habits for staying "Well Past Forty" by typing the phrase **wellpastforty** into a search engine. Try it.

For his R&R, Dave enjoys the Vitamin D offered by Southern California weather while rowing competitively or trail-hiking, or sharing sea stories with his service pals and US Naval Academy alumni. He also writes academic papers about 21st century workplaces and knowledge workers as most valuable players.

KABOOMER: Thriving and Striving into your 90s was written for a subset of millions of beneficiary baby boomers, keying on Dave's personal experiences and professional expertise. He is a Master Fitness Trainer, an award-winning adjunct professor, a proud grandfather, world-ranked oarsman, and a communications expert. Many moons ago, he was an Eagle Scout, an Outstanding College Athlete of America (1975), and a decorated naval officer in Cold War days. Yes, he is a mid-cycle baby boomer. But more, he chooses to do those "little bits extra" to better his chances to party past 90. This book is his "talk the walk" almanac to help many others on their own journeys past Medicare age. Be a KABOOMER too!

Acknowledgements

Labors of love like this specialty non-fiction work are seldom solitary. *KABOOMER: Thriving and Striving into Your 90s* was indeed a Book Launcher team effort. This book compiles many influences in my life, sharing with you my many lessons learned. My "**7S formula**" combines the influence and wisdom of passionate and purposeful people, my own body of work, and credible references to help you sustain healthy habits to party past 90. Without these ingredients, your Koach's recipe would better serve average baby boomers, not our female and male demographic peers who are determined KABOOMERs. Applying these ingredients and influences, I KABOOM.

I trust that you will, too, adding years to your life and life to your years.

I am particularly grateful to my New England forebears and parents, to my wonderful wife, Mary, and to my collegiate rowing coach, Carl Ullrich, who is of the Greatest Generation known to mankind. Two incredible kids helped make this Koach who he is. True thanks to my artist, Austeja. High kudos to Uncle Sam and his extraordinary soldiers, sailors, airmen, and marines, plus their dependents who serve US every day. I proudly tip my naval cover to Academy colleagues, "flower children" classmates, and to my shipmates for the tangible and intangible gifts they proffered to me. And to my many hundreds of students and clients: Gracias! KABOOM.

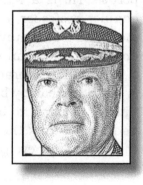

CPSIA information can be obtained
at www.ICGtesting.com
Printed in the USA
BVHW031012300922
648388BV00003B/7

9 780578 891125

The Jerome Conspiracy